JEREMIAH D. TIPTON, Ph.D

D1170325

THE
N-of-1
CHALLENGE

A Real-Life Guide
to Optimizing
Individual Health

Cover Design: Kurt Richmond, kurt.richmond@oddballdesignz.com

Inside Layout: Ljiljana Pavkov

Printed in the United States

ISBN: 978-1-7330311-0-3 (paperback)

ISBN: 978-1-7330311-1-0 (eBook)

Dedicated to my sister and father,
both of whom left us last year.
To celebrating with you,
our accomplishments.

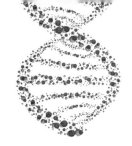

TABLE OF CONTENTS

THE
N-of-1
CHALLENGE

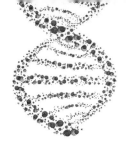

ACKNOWLEDGEMENTS

Thank you to Jim White from Old Baldy Photography for taking and preparing the pictures for the figures in this book. Your contribution is greatly appreciated.

I would like to thank Jade Skinner, a local Yoga instructor for her education and conversation on the different forms of yoga.

I also want to acknowledge Devin Tipton for his contributions towards the design of the book cover.

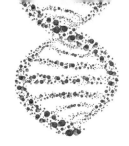

INTRODUCTION

Life can be challenging, especially when we are not treating ourselves well. I don't believe that we choose to be unhealthy - it's more that we need to be mindful of the changes with our body as we age. We also may need to make adjustments in our lifestyle to stay healthy. In my opinion, one of the biggest challenges that we fight in today's society is having enough time to take care of ourselves. Especially for those with careers and a few children to raise, finding time for self-care may be incredibly difficult. However, with all the demands in our lives, we must still schedule time for ourselves. We need to take care of our core strength. We also need to pay attention to what we are eating. Both, a simple 30-minute workout each day, and watching what we eat can make monumental changes in our overall health.

During our life's journey, we can tend to stop paying attention to our health and the lifestyles that we live. If we are not mindful, we can let ourselves slip into a health slump. At one point during my life, I fell into a health slump. Some of this book is based on what I learned while working towards my goals and a healthy lifestyle. During my health slump, I had reached the point where I ate whatever I wanted, neglected my core-strength, and had spent many years just working hard at my career.

I was not living a healthy lifestyle and I was definitely not paying attention to my overall health. Over time, my body had begun to deteriorate, and I was well on my way to becoming overweight and pre-diabetic. I woke up one day with continued chronic pain in my back and joints and decided that I was going to make changes. It took a couple of years to get back on track -this included losing 55 pounds to get back to my healthy living weight. Thus, this book is a discussion on three important topics of health: nutrition, core strength, and what I will call mind-space, which is akin to mental health management.

For my background, I have performed research in the life sciences and biotechnology industries for over fifteen years on all sorts of diseases. Some of these diseases include brain cancer (glioblastoma), Alzheimer's disease, and tropical diseases. I have worked on all sorts of research related to drug discovery and molecular biology. Along with some of my personal recovery story, I present some of the most recent information with regards to obesity and the link to diabetes research. During the book, one of the questions that we want to answer is: Why is it important to change our lifestyles and diets?

Even with my understanding of human disease and the numerous projects I have worked on, I still fell into a health slump. I worked hard at my career but did not take care of myself. As we go through this book, we will follow some of the factors that contributed to my slip in health. As well, we will discuss what actions I finally settled upon to help me regain my full capacity.

Life is a marathon, not a sprint.

This book intends to discuss nutrition, core strength, and mind-space with regard to obesity and its connection to diseases such as prediabetes and Type 2 diabetes. This book lays out several aspects that are important for our health that are *within our control*, including what we eat, our physical activity level, and our mental health.

The goal of this book is not to replace your visit to the doctor; it is to make your doctor visits better. We live in an era of information overload and at times it can be difficult to determine what is helpful. I hope that this book brings you some guidance while sailing through the sea of information. This book is also intended to present a *sustainability mindset* with regard to nutrition, core strength, and mind-space. When speaking with one of my colleagues about this book, he used the analogy of a three-legged stool. When all three legs are working, we are on solid ground. Even if the ground is uneven, the stool can handle it. Whatever happens during life, you will have the ability to maintain balance. Of course, this is not true if one leg is weak or missing entirely.

As we age, our minds and bodies change. At different ages, we require different plans for nutrition, core strength, and mind-space management. Practices that worked for us in our twenties, in terms of diet and exercise, will not work later in life. As well, our mental pressure and aptitudes change. But this is what's great about being human—we have the ability to adapt to ever-changing environments and needs. Those who can adapt and change to fit their environments are often most successful during life's struggles.

No matter what stage you are at in life—your age, sex, demographic, or special needs—you have an *individual optimal lifestyle* plan that is dependent on your current and future bodily needs.

This book is designed to be a short guide on how to think about your own personal health plan and what you, as an individual, need to do. In the spirit of this philosophy, this book is intended to help you understand the concept of the "N-of-1 Challenge" and your health. Each of us are unique with regard to our needs for improved nutrition, core strength, and mind-space management. As you go through the following chapters in this book, it has been broken this book into 4 parts. The first part is in regard to awareness, habits, and the "N-of-1 Challenge" concept. Also in Part 1, I include stories of real people that changed their diets and lifestyles. Normally, this type of section would be left for later in the book. These stories are at the beginning of the book because I want you to see that change is possible. I also want you to see that people can improve their lifestyles and health for different reasons.

Part 2 is a discussion about nutrition as it relates to obesity, carbohydrates, and disease. This section is designed to increase awareness of obesity-related diseases such as prediabetes and Type 2 diabetes. I include some basic tools that take a look at the number of carbohydrates you are consuming and how to scale back.

Part 3 discusses core strength, mobility, and physical activity. Your current level of health will dictate where you need to start with new core strength training. You may need to start with stretching if mobility and chronic pain are issues.

Part 4 is related to mental health. Here, we look at ways to manage what I call "mind-space," a critical but sometimes overlooked element of any healthy lifestyle. In this section of the book, I discuss several topics related to mental health management of mind-space. We will discuss meditation, yoga, prayer, and community. As well, we will have an interview with a holistic care practitioner. Holistic care includes looking at the human as a whole and I believe that the basic building blocks for this type of care includes nutrition, core strength, and mind-space management.

As a reminder, if you have had major injuries during your lifetime, please consult your doctor before adding routines to your lifestyle (especially high-intensity cardio or weightlifting activities). Anytime you engage in new physical activities, it is best to consult a licensed coach or specialist. Also, listen to your doctor. Our goal is to heal ourselves from injury, not further injure ourselves. Proper supervision and coaching can be necessary.

Another goal of this book is to give you tools and information so that you can reach what the doctor and specialist prescribe. Each of us is unique with regard to our needs for nutrition, core strength, and mind-space management. As you journey through life, you are the only one who can decide for yourself that *obtaining a healthy lifestyle is important*. No one else is going to do this for you. And remember - if it sounds like an excuse, it probably is.

Sometimes, we devote excessive amounts of hard work into improving an aspect of our health, only to revert to old habits (i.e. the "Yo-Yo Effect," you lose 10 pounds, then gain 15 back). This book is *not* about offering an easy fix. We are not talking about overnight changes; we are talking about changing habits to change our lifestyles to improve our overall health. Your current level of physical and mental health will dictate the amount of time it will take to get back to a manageable lifestyle. Your body will let you know. Awareness is Step 1. After I became fully aware of what I needed to improve my health, it took me four years to fully reach my long-term goals. But I did meet my goals and you will too.

PART 1:

AWARENESS, HABITS, AND THE
N-OF-1 CHALLENGE

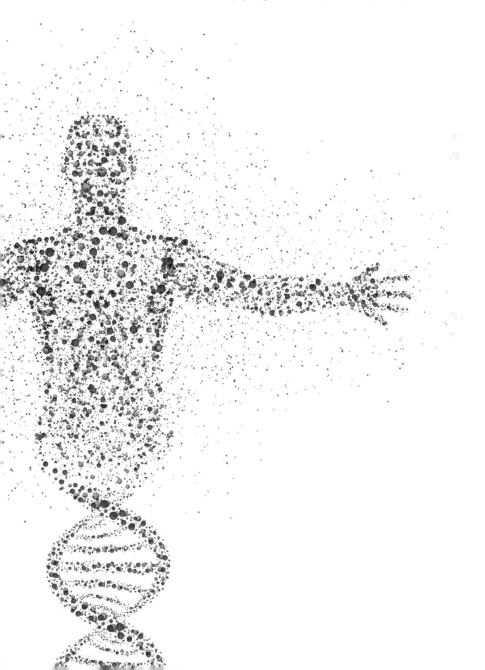

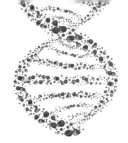

CHAPTER 1:

THE BASICS OF AWARENESS, HABITS, AND OVERUSE INJURIES

A habit is typically defined as an action we perform with regularity— often without much thought given to the process. We are creatures of habit, and many of us require normal routines to live day-to-day. Habits can be long-term, short-term, or intentionally shaped and formed to meet our desires within the framework of our environment.

There have been volumes of books written on the importance of habit-forming behaviors and suggestions, some of which have been included in the reference section of this book (**REF 1, 2, 3**). I believe that you understand habits and habit formation; building upon cumulative knowledge is valuable during this journey. I also trust that you may know half or most of the information in this book. If you don't, I hope to help you with some enlightening thoughts. This book is about taking what you already know about habit-forming behaviors and applying it to what you may need to do to improve your health.

This book is designed to discuss the three basics of health as related to *nutrition, core strength, and mind-space*. We also want to design actionable plans to help reach the goals that we set. Many of the suggestions in this book come from my personal experiences, as well as biomedical research that I was part of or reviewed. In regard to my experiences,

I already understood habits and performed biomedical research, but I still had to sit down and make a health plan that made sense - I had aged, and what was good for me during my late 20s did not work for me in my late 30s.

As discussed in the introduction, the way we treat ourselves in regard to our health dictates how healthy we feel. If one of the three main topics —nutrition, physical activity, or mind-space—is not in alignment, we will not feel fully well. And if one of the areas is not balanced, it can cause problems with the other two.

Very often we have habits that we believe are acceptable. Often, these habits are related to our health. How many people have said: "I'll start my diet tomorrow" or, "It's OK to have that extra piece of cake" or, "My back is just going to hurt, it's just the way it is," or "I can never give up bread at dinner." There are so many daily thoughts that we have that are poor rationalizations.

However, I am not sure that a poor choice is always due to a lack of willpower. Food can have addictive properties. Also, when it comes to working out and eating healthy, many people "fall off the wagon" during the winter months and the holidays. Gym memberships spike in January, and many people donate money to the gym for the rest of the year - I was guilty of this at one point during my health slip cycles. Or, we have long-term sugar consumption issues (specifically, added sugar products) because of how accessible those products have become. Even though we have "human tendencies," if we are in tune with our body and mind, our awareness of these cycles can be challenged. Habits and cycles that we may have maintained our whole lives may be difficult to change. One way to look at a our choices with regard to nutrition, physical activity, or mind-space is: *Could I injure myself with this choice?* Another way to look at it is: *Am I 'overusing' this?* The overuse could be a food, an activity, or a thought pattern. I believe that if you are overusing anything—sitting all day, eating too many carbs, or fixating on problems that keep you up at night—that you will injure yourself in some way. What sort of overuse habits do you possibly have in your life?

Overuse Injuries and the Link to the Three Basics of Optimal Health

Throughout this book, I will share my journey and recovery from "overuse" injuries. I have found that overuse is a common theme among the current lifestyles we tend to see in society. While consulting with other subject-matter experts for this project and book, I found that overuse can be applied to three topics of discussion:

(1) Physical Activity: overuse (or underuse) of a muscle group or joint
(2) Diet and Nutrition: overuse of different foods that cause obesity or illness
(3) Mind-Space: overuse of the mind to the point of burnout

1. Physical Activity

Overuse injuries are most easily recognized by the presence of physical pain; a muscle or joint causes pain when we move it or perform a certain activity. Overuse in this sense can occur simply from sitting too long at a desk, causing our muscles to literally 'shorten' during several years of neglect. Overuse can also be associated with working out too hard, thus injuring ourselves. Overuse can arise from any sort of repetitive motions that we do during the day. Chapter 8 discusses this topic more in-depth, including what you can do to mitigate this problem.

When I spoke with Alyssa Stewart about physical therapy, one of the subject matter experts who will be interviewed in Chapter 8, she said that 90% of her patients' issues stem from muscles being out of balance, thus creating pain. Classic examples include back or knee pain arising from a muscle pulling on a joint or a muscle group simply not being in balance. With proper training over time, Alyssa could conservatively help patients with pain and teach them what needs to be done to maintain core strength. This means that you may be able to treat your pain through physical therapy treatments—without the need for surgery or medication. Does avoiding the need to take medication sound appealing? Part 3 of this book is dedicated to topics related to physical activity.

2. Diet and Nutrition

Other overuse injuries can be related to diet and nutrition. If we were to frame diet into this concept, I believe that obesity, prediabetes, and Type 2 diabetes fall into the "overuse" category. In Chapter 6, I list statistics and provide important information for obesity, prediabetes, and Type 2 diabetes that is very eye-opening. If we think of obesity as an overuse injury, perhaps we can begin to understand why we need to stop consuming so much "sugar water" and high-calorie food. Obesity is the effect of energy storage (aka fat) for future use. If we keep gaining weight because of our diet, are we not overusing food?

Obesity is a major risk factor for several diseases, including prediabetes and Type 2 diabetes. Correctly stated, obesity creates a situation where our bodies have a hard time regulating the sugar in our blood. Thus, we have more sugar in our blood, all the time. This, in turn, creates a situation where our bodies create more insulin—the substance needed to help transport and use sugar throughout our bodies. Eventually, our body cannot keep up with insulin production because of the high amounts of sugar in the blood. Thus, we get high amounts of sugar in our blood, and the insulin system breaks down or can only work to a certain level.

Please note that I am not saying that sugar is inherently bad, but that *overuse* of sugar is bad. We need sugar for proper brain function and energy. Chapters 4, 5, and 6 continue the discussion of sugar overuse with regard to diseases and risk factors.

Unlike the easily identified physical pain that results from physical injuries, a nutrition overuse injury can sneak up on us over long periods of time. It is much easier to lose 10 pounds that it is 20. It's really easy to gain 10 to 20 pounds. It's really hard to lose 30 pounds. The time frames for all of these scenarios are very different. The level of difficulty to lose 30 pounds at 40 years old is much different than that at 30.

3. Mind-Space

Another example of an overuse injury is the classic mental burnout due to stress, work, and generally not sleeping. Although stress is not a major topic of this book, mind-space is. We don't want to fix the stress—the stress is not the problem. This process is about how the mind is managed so that the stress does not manage us.

For this book and discussion, mind-space refers to the amount of thoughts that you can have, subconsciously or consciously. Mind-space is not about being happy all the time. Often, this topic gets confused as a quest for some sort of emotional utopia—the idea of achieving a mindset where "everything is going to be great." I describe "mind-space" as being more related to how we manage our thoughts than it is about managing a feeling. Feelings are the result of how we manage our minds. Stress is a result of how we manage our minds. The mind-space concept is essential to managing the habits that we form. Our minds can become burnt out if we are not paying attention—just like our nutrition and physical health. I have often found that the mind follows down the path of negativity along with poor nutrition or lack of physical activity.

Mind-space can also be looked at like it is a muscle. It needs to be worked out. Just like there are those born with innately great physical gifts (professional athletes), there are those born with innately great minds for handling stress. As with all things in life, we all have certain work to do on our minds, just like we lift weights for strength. Part 4 of this book reviews different mental exercises and practices to help with mind-space management.

Nurture vs. Nature

In the previous section, we looked at habits and overuse injuries and connected that conversation to the three main topics of this book: nutrition, core strength, and mind-space. Most overuse injuries are dependent on what we have in our control—the food we eat, the physical activity we perform, and our mental health practice. If your daily habits are causing your body harm, then consider creating a new habit or taking a new action. These actions are put in the category of "nurture"—they can be controlled by self. This is simple logic. However, if this is such simple logic, then why are 1 in 3 Americans prediabetic?

Nature

To continue this discussion, let's look at some of the major factors that influence our health, then relate them back to our three main topics and our major themes.

- Genetics and Heritage
- Diet (Nutrition)
- Physical Activity
- Mental and Emotional Stress
- Environment (i.e., Pollution)

For the purposes of this book, we are not going to discuss genetic factors as the reason for "slipping in health". We are going to consider things like diet, physical activity, and mental health.

We live in what is called the "Genomics Era," meaning we can measure someone's predisposition to certain conditions and diseases through genetic testing. Of course, this does not mean that people will always get the disease based on a genetic test. To be honest, we don't always know why a disease does or does not happen, even if there is a predisposition, or lack thereof. However, there are several great scientific studies that point us in the correct direction for different diseases or even define them. Nature is very complex, and the exact answer is not always available as to why a disease occurs. As we sometimes say in biomedical research, "Nature does not reveal her answers easily."

Of course, we cannot ignore genetics completely. Genetic factors can help us make choices for how we should change our lifestyles. For example, if you were to sit down with a nutrition specialist, genetics and/or family history should be part of the conversation. If you have a family history of Type 2 diabetes, how far can you trace it? Parents? Siblings? Great-great-grandparents? A genetic (or apparent genetic) predisposition for Type 2 diabetes should be considered when deciding on an optimal diet and workout plan. It's also important to realize you can still get Type 2 diabetes *without* having a genetic disposition; everyone who is obese has a predisposition for pre- and Type 2 diabetes.

A genetic predisposition means that you have a higher *chance* of a certain disease developing. It does not always mean that it *will* happen.

We cannot control our genetics, but we *can* control what we eat, our physical activities, and how we manage our mental health. We are going to focus on habits and re-forming good habits. Our genetic programming will not do this for us. We have to perform the tasks needed to improve our health. If you have a test that says you have a predisposition to a disease, learn about the risk factors so that you can avoid (or add) certain foods or activities that will increase the likelihood of the disease happening.

Nurture

Results from genetic tests do not consider environmental interactions and their effect on health. With my skill set, I can take someone's urine or blood and tell them all sorts of useful information about their body and health. But will that information help someone who doesn't *want* to change their behaviors to become healthier? I love technology, genomics, and the life sciences. Modern biomedical research is very powerful, often revealing all sorts of highly beneficial Information. But just because we can measure someone's genetic predisposition to a disease and current health profile, that does not mean that we are in tune with what the body is telling us. Another goal of this book is to provide you with the tools to get in tune with your body and what it is telling you.

Doctors can only make decisions based on test results, what you say, and how you respond. Doctors can only help based on your feedback. One of the biggest frustrations for doctors in modern medicine and patient care is lack of compliance with prescriptions and proper feedback. This can sometimes be linked with prideful behaviors. Pride can be one of the most destructive forces preventing people from improvement. It prevents us from listening to our doctors and or specialist. Many people go to their doctor and receive results that are not exactly good, say, high cholesterol. The doctor says, "You need to change your diet and perform physical exercise." If the patient is full of pride, then it is difficult to get through to them. These are the people that reach a full diagnosis of a disease -they are too stubborn to listen.

There are also those that initially do what the doctor says, then over time, they stop performing the prescribed tasks. This book may be best for those that believe what the doctor is saying. If this describes your situation, this book looks to stop the Yo-Yo effect. Over time, this group of people has simply not formed the habits needed to stay in compliance with the advice and prescription.

With regard to nurturing mind-space, if you are not committed to a sustainable mindset, you may follow your doctor's prescription, get to a healthy point, then go back to previous behaviors. You'll get sick again, go see the doctor and start the cycle over again, costing more money to you and the health care system. Do you like wasting money? Does this sound familiar? We are what we eat, and we are the habits that we form. It is up to you to understand what your body is telling you and to do what needs to be done. I personally think that the digital age has brought with it a lack of the virtue of *"Knowing Thyself."* This book is designed to help cultivate this philosophy as well.

As we age, we simply do not have the same healing powers we did when we were younger. As you read this book, you will see how important mind-space truly is and how it is linked to nutrition and physical activity. No one can stop the aging process, but we can all still live a sustainable lifestyle. Sustainability can have many meanings in today's society. In this book, we will apply the sustainability concept to nutrition, physical activity, and mind-space.

To reiterate, I believe that most people already know how to improve their health; it's inherent to our success as a human race. Depending on where we are in life, in terms of age, weight, and diet, it can be very difficult to know where to start—especially if we have been treating ourselves poorly for many years. This brings us to a framework for action items and goals in this book. We all have our own **"N-of-1 Challenge"** that can be optimized to reach our personal lifestyle.

The **Challenge** is to find your balance in the three main topics described in this book: nutrition, core strength, and mind-space. The only person who knows where you are with your health is *you*. So, what do I mean by "N-of-1 Challenge"? I will cover this topic in the next chapter.

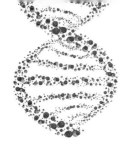

CHAPTER 2:

THE N-OF-1 CHALLENGE

In biomedical research, the term "N-of-1" usually refers to a single patient in a clinical trial of some sort. The consideration is that the patient is the sole unit of observation during that study. During the investigation, the study will look at the effectiveness or the side-effect profiles (aka "efficacy") of different interventions or medicines. Thus, this normally refers to the study of drug interactions within the body of a single individual (**REF 4**).

It is not standard practice to look at the effects of drugs on a single individual for research purposes. Normally, we recruit hundreds or thousands of patients to participate in a clinical study. Once the study is designed and completed, we use statistical programs to find trends related to a particular disease or condition. The observed trends help researchers and medical doctors make decisions on which drugs or interventions to pursue. Collecting large data sets on clinical trials has been very powerful for finding the mechanisms of different diseases and new drug treatments.

I have worked in research fields that rely on "big data" - i.e. sorting through enormous amounts of data to find trends to help make decisions. The current mindset is that we should rely on big data for decision-making, all the time. But in my opinion, relying solely on big data can mask certain important information related to individuals. Big data is associated with collecting data on bulk populations—hundreds or thousands of people—and identifying trends based on the results. The term "N-of-1" is associated with looking at and treating someone as an individual. For the purposes of this book, we are looking at an individual's diet, core strength, and mental health.

There is a growing body of evidence that unique results may be missing from big-data analysis because the experiment is designed to compare individuals from large clinical studies. Not to be understated - big-data has helped us advance toward solutions for health care and has provided solutions for many other industries. More recently, however, I have adopted the concept of N-of-1 when it comes to health and lifestyle, as opposed to just looking at big data.

I believe that if we all take the time to understand that we all have unique health and lifestyle needs, we can make the improvements we require. This has driven me back to looking at individuals, not just at big-data or at data points in a study. We need to accept that each one of us may have different needs in the areas of nutrition, physical activity, and mind-space. The N-of-1 concept (in regard to this book) means that *you are your own health and nutrition experiment.* Naturally, your optimal level of nutritional needs, physical activity, and mind-space practices may be different than those of your friends, family, and colleagues.

The N-of-1 Challenge involves setting goals in all three areas of life—nutrition, core strength, and mind-space. We can collect as much information as we like, but if we don't put proper effort into improvement, nothing will change for the better. Parts 2, 3, and 4 of this book continue to discuss each of the three areas separately. Throughout this book, I will present examples of goals that can help you reach new levels in your N-of-1 Challenge. Only you know what is needed for your N-of-1 optimal health. Only you know how you feel and what makes you feel really alive.

That is what makes this a *challenge.* Simply measuring metrics and consuming information will not help you improve your life. You have to reach your goals. You have to challenge yourself. You have to set your own N-of-1 Challenge.

The N-of-1 Challenge and Nutrition

There are, of course, certain base foods that all humans need to consume in order to stay healthy. With that said, perhaps the start of an N-of-1 Challenge is to just eat less food. Consume less. On the other hand, the nutrition aspect of your N-of-1 Challenge may be the most difficult of the three categories. An initial example of something to think about for your Challenge: To what foods do you have sensitivity, intolerance, or allergies?

Many people have some sort of food sensitivity or intolerance. Are you sensitive to wheat, nightshades, peanuts, shellfish, etc.? Some allergies, such as peanuts and shellfish, are easy to understand—you swell up, and your body goes into a very bad allergic/inflammatory response. A wheat or nightshade sensitivity, on the other hand, might be much subtler. You eat the food and don't really feel that well, but because you don't have a strong allergic reaction, the sensitivity or intolerance goes unnoticed.

Personally, I have several food sensitivities and intolerances that I have identified over time with "addition/subtraction dieting." This is when we subtract (or don't eat) a certain food that is known to possibly cause allergies and/or inflammation. Then, you simply pay attention to how your body feels or reacts to the subtraction or addition of various foods. Sometimes, you may even initially go through withdrawal-type symptoms because of food addiction. A quick personal example, I have a wheat sensitivity. When I identified this sensitivity, it caused the largest shift in my diet. I simply cannot have bread, pasta or many types of beer. It *will* make me sick to varying degrees of exposure and type of food. Thus, I have adjusted my nutritional habits to reflect this reality. I have found that a balanced diet, lacking empty carbs and added sugar, works best for me. As well, the elimination of wheat from my diet resulted in less inflammation in my joints. I feel amazing most of the time now.

A second nutrition challenge is to rein in the overuse of refined sugar and carbohydrates. The nutrition part of this book is mostly about this topic. The overuse of food leads to obesity, thus creating all sorts of health risks. Later in this book, I cover risk factors associated with obesity. Do you consume too much refined sugar and or empty carbohydrates? Obesity can lead to diseases like prediabetes and Type 2 diabetes. Chapters 5 and 6 are dedicated to nutrition and diet; we will discuss these topics in more detail there.

Over time, I have naturally progressed to what is commonly known now as a paleo diet. To me, this diet is based on the philosophy of eating what humans ate before all of the processed foods that we eat now. I follow a "practical" Paleo diet—veggies, fruits, meat, a minimal amount of added-sugar foods, and a highly regulated intake of carbs from food such as rice to sweet potatoes. I say "practical" because, well, what's the use of living without cheesecake sometimes? I personally don't always agree with what people call paleo foods, but I do know how my body reacts to foods that have been processed. As we go on, we are only going to focus on excess added sugar and "empty" carbohydrate foods.

I don't believe that any single "diet" is best for everyone. For example, there are those out there that claim that a vegan diet is *the only way to go*. For some, this will work as their diet plan. But I don't think everyone should adopt any plan until they understand what they actually need.

To move into the next discussion on core strength, I don't think everyone should become a powerlifter. To be honest, if you want to become a powerlifter, this book is probably not for you. If you would like to become a powerlifter for your N-of-1 Challenge, the goals for diet and exercise will be different than that described in this book. This book is more about the basics of nutrition and core strength, rather than advice on advanced training.

The N-of-1 Challenge for Core Strength and Physical Activity

How many years have you lacked physical activity or core strength training? The choice of your physical activity for your N-of 1 Challenge will be dependent on your current activity, past activity, and possible overuse injuries. It will also be based on other acute injuries suffered during your lifetime.

As you reach your personal N-of-1 Challenge goals, you will improve and reach new levels of core strength. You may reach a core strength that you remember from your youth. You may even reach unrealized levels of mobility and general well-being. Also, the best part of core strength training is that there are so many physical activities that you can choose from! In my opinion, this can be fun and less grueling than a diet change. You will also find people who have similar interests in physical activities and training. Remember, these activities should be fun! Chapters 8, 9, and 10 are dedicated to core strength concepts, as well as different physical activity plans.

For my own story, my knees are not in the best shape and I really cannot perform high impact training. This is more related to ligament and cartilage damage, as opposed to having muscles out of balance. I have learned how to keep my muscles in balance so that I do not create unnecessary stress on them. Often, they ache if I don't properly stretch or if I perform high-impact training. This issue is from numerous minor sports injuries due to a "reckless abandon" style of play. I have learned what I can do to keep my body healthy so that I don't create new injuries. Thus, when I was working to find my personal N-of-1, jogging and power lifting turned out to be poor options. It turned out that cycling and a light-weight / high rep training were much better choices.

As my health improved the last 4 years of re-training I added new activities as I reached different goals. I had to add new stretches to my regimen to counterbalance the "shortening" of muscles due to cycling. This forced me into a more rigorous "long stretch routine" during the mornings or sometimes evenings depending on my schedule. Since the start of my recovery from my health slip, I now work out 2 to 4 times a week, along with cycling 3 to 4 days a week. The workouts or only take 35 to 55 minutes a week.

Also, learning about mobility and core strength helped me improve my health rapidly. Before selecting cycling as my cardio workout, my N-of-1 was to walk 1 to 3 miles on the beach. Before walks on the beach, I had to perform physical training on my back and hip muscles in order to rebalance the muscle groups I had neglected and overused. I took time to learn about the specific muscle groups that I was working on. I became re-connected with my body and understood the source of the chronic pain. This was an opportunity to notice how all of my individual muscles and joints felt as I fixed what needed to be improved.

Thus, prior to making changes in my life, I had reached a point of chronic pain. My physical activity was just walking on the beach. Now, 5 years later, I work out 3 days a week and cycle 50 to 100 miles per week. After 5 years of continuous stretching, I have become more flexible. I made stretching a routine and a new habit. I did not just get up and charge into the day, I made time for myself. For the first time in my life, I have been able to almost put my palms flat on the ground while performing a hamstring stretch. Before this, I could only stretch to the point where my fingertips were at the lower part of my shin.

This is a path to learning how to connect with *your* body and to understand what you are improving. If you need a coach or a trainer, plan to get one. Coaches can be pivotal for helping you with the re-formation of goals and habits to reach your own N-of-1 Challenge.

The N-of-1 Challenge and Mind-Space Management

At the beginning of this book, we discussed habits and the poor rationalization of the habits we may currently have. The discussion earlier in the book is the basis for improving our mind-space management. While changing our diet and working to improve our core strength, we also need to make sure that we are managing our mental health. This management has 2 major themes in this book.

The first is paying attention to the habits that we have now and new habit formation. I referenced several books that are solely dedicated to habit forming behaviors **(REF 1, 2, 3)**. These books include *The Power of Now: A Guide to Spiritual Enlightenment* by Eckhart Tolle; *The Power of Habit: Why We Do What We Do in Life and Business* by Charles Duhigg; and *Mini Habits: Smaller Habits, Bigger Results* by Stephen Guise. I ask that you review one of these books when you get a chance. I prefer the book written by Eckhart Tolle.

The second major theme for mental-space management is mental burnout because of overuse and stress. In Part 4 of this book, I draw on other analogies to try and make you think about mind-space and mental health in other terms. I try to quantify mind-space in the same way that we would count calories or count the number of hours we perform physical activity. Many of us don't put a value on our mind-space and the amount of energy that we really have to give.

Probably the most important concept to understand is that over time, we age, our bodies change, and we have different needs. We often don't change our habits to match our needs. This is why I have broken the book down into the three important areas of life. The only constant during life is change. Those who are most adaptable to change will survive the longest. However, on the other side of the coin, there are constants that we can maintain in life to help manage these changes. Habit-forming behaviors are essential to managing nutrition, core strength, and mind-space.

With health—as with most things in life—people only tend to address an issue if there is a major problem. I feel that this is one of the biggest problems in society—the lack of preventative maintenance. We practice sick care not healthcare. If you don't change the oil in your car, what will happen? What happens if you don't change the filter on your air conditioner? What if you did not perform basic maintenance on the machines you rely on in your daily life? Why do we treat machinery better than the way we treat our bodies and minds? Instead of creating the drama of a problem-solution pair, why not spend time on sustainability?

Good and poor habits are more often learned behaviors. We are all human. An important aspect of mental health and mind-space management is that no one is perfect—so forgive yourself first. All we need to do is re-form habits that will lead to a healthier lifestyle. Pay attention to what your body is telling you. Follow your body's inner wisdom and its innate ability to heal itself.

Over the next 3 parts of this book, I will continue to expand on what we covered so far. However, before getting into a discussion on the three topics of this book, I want to share some stories with you. These stories are different examples of how people achieved healthy lifestyles through their own N-of-1 Challenges.

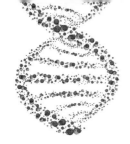

CHAPTER 3:

HOW OTHER PEOPLE CHANGED THEIR LIFESTYLES

In most books of this type, this sort of chapter would be left for later. But rather than define concepts and prescribe action items, I would like you to see where other people were with their health, what their tipping point was, and what they did to change their lifestyles. There is nothing more powerful than real stories from people that were able to make real changes.

In this chapter, I also share my personal story. You will find additional stories about my health slump and recovery throughout this book. I have interviewed several individuals who have made major lifestyle changes in the three key areas discussed in this book. My hope is that this book reaches many people that need it and that we will be able to share more stories in the future. Each of these individual stories reveals that we can be successful and reach our goals if we choose to work toward them.

We all age, and our bodies deteriorate—especially if we don't put effort into counteracting the effects. Life is a journey and if we are not paying attention, we can let things go or fall into a health slump. No one *intentionally* falls into a health slump, but it is easy to do. Life has its ebbs and flows, and at times, we can find ourselves "out-of-shape," whether it be mentally, physically, or both.

Aging is rough on the body and mind. One of the most common changes as we age is our **metabolism**. Most of us ate whatever we wanted until our 20s or 30s. Our metabolism continues to slow down over time, but you can combat that. The goal is to adapt to our bodies' needs as they change over time. Of course, there are no absolutes. All we can really do is increase the likelihood of living a long, fruitful life.

There are no secrets when it comes to food and nutrition. It is *what we choose* to eat and *how we choose* to live our lives that makes the difference.

My "Health Slump" Story

At one point during my life, I had been working 70-hour weeks, traveling all over the South, not sleeping, and eating whatever I wanted. I enjoyed this life, but it took a toll on me. Prior to this phase, I had performed research on a variety of medically relevant topics and worked on developing some very cool biomedical tests. For over 10 years during this period, I was easily working 60 to 70-hour weeks as well. When you are "all-in" on your research, you don't really think about anything else. On top of those 70-hour weeks, I pushed myself hard to always have fun on the weekends, and I pushed to stay in the loop in my social life. "You can sleep when you're dead" was my lifestyle mentality. In the end, I worked this lifestyle for over 15 years, if not longer.

About 6 years ago I realized that I was 55 pounds overweight! My body and mind were not in tune with my real needs. I had watched myself continue to make poor decisions and it was time to make a change. I was only worried about my clients, my company, and my career. Then I woke up one day and asked, "What the hell am I doing?!"

I had pushed myself too hard, too far, and for too long - a top performer. I was in chronic pain from overuse injuries and was eating all sorts unhealth, empty carbohydrate foods. I never really had a sweet tooth growing up and never ate much sugar in general, but I was getting most of my calories from eating all sorts of food during meetings with clients or drinking beer with friends on the weekends. My body had changed, but my mind had not.

It feels great to be able to say that I did eventually get everything under control. I lost those 55 pounds and normalized my diet and physical activities. I also started to meditate so that I could calm my mind. It took me about 4 years to get fully "back to normal."

After realizing that I had neglected my mind and body for at least a decade, I tried several "Work-out Startups," but nothing stuck. I ate whatever I wanted, whenever I wanted, and ignored the food sensitivities that I had developed over time. It wasn't until I was physically and mentally exhausted that I finally did something about it—like most people. Specifically, for me—with my knowledge and the industry I work in—there was no reason for me to allow that to happen!

Key Point: *Don't beat yourself up. It is not productive. Self-destructive thoughts are never helpful while trying to improve your health.*

Personally, I found that the nutrition and physical activity portions of my health were easier to improve than my mind-space. Nutrition and physical activity improvements came easily when I just paid attention and put the work in. This may be because I lack a sweet tooth for nutrition and was an athlete earlier in life for physical activity.

I found that mind-space and meditation were more difficult for me to work on. Those parts took several years, probably because of the creative, over-active, analytical mind that I was born with. For me, it's hard to drop out of a thought pattern or stop working on a project until it's at full completion. I have achieved great improvements in mind-space management, and meditation has been very helpful.

Certain people will need to work harder in some areas than others. But we all need to start somewhere. As mentioned earlier, I interviewed several people who changed their lifestyles. They all found their own optimal lifestyle through their N-of-1 Challenge. They made their own challenges and reached their goals. Some people needed extra coaching and a support system. While on their journey, they did not know they were working toward their own N-of-1 Challenge.

For each of the following interviews, I asked the same set of questions. Below, I have filled out the questionnaire with my own answers as an introduction to this section.

At the end of this book, in Chapter 13, I have included a blank set of questions for you to answer if you like.

Recovery Story 1 – Jeremiah Tipton, Author

1) While growing up, what sort of diet did you have, and what sorts of athletic activities did you participate in (high school through college)? Can you describe your diet from that time?

In high school, I played baseball during the spring. I tried basketball (I was never really good at it) and football. I ended up getting migraines my junior year, so I stopped playing football.

During college, I played all of the intermural sports (flag football, softball, ultimate frisbee, inner tube water polo, etc.) However, after college, I no longer played sports and really didn't go to the gym. During graduate school and during my last two years there, I really did not play many sports. I spent most of my time in the lab or reading/writing at a desk.

While I was growing up, we had fresh, frozen, and canned vegetables. We did not consume sweets or have soda products around. Most of our extra sugar came from Kool-Aid. Our carb intake was from pasta (most nights) and potatoes. We also always had fresh fruit around to eat for snacks. During college, I ate whatever I wanted (and drank more beer than I should have). It was a very unhealthy diet. However, I did continue to stay away from candy and soda products. I remember living on fifty-cent hamburgers or two-for-one pizzas for $10 or nachos from 7-Eleven. Eating properly as a poor college student was very difficult.

2) What were the factors (or reasons) that contributed to your loss in overall health?

My decline in health probably started toward the end of graduate school. I was not eating healthy, I was not exercising, and, if you have ever worked through an advanced higher-education program, you know that it can be very mentally taxing. After my advanced degree, I realized that I was slipping, so I tried to go to the gym, but it was not as fun as playing team sports. My diet had probably been terrible since I started college.

As I aged, I had more and more problems with my back and chronic pain. I had seen doctors and chiropractors, but it did not seem to help in the long run. I was mentally fixated purely on my research and work. I was ignoring what my body was trying to tell me. I had become a workaholic.

This went on for at least five more years before I found myself in Dr. Dex Alvarez's office in great pain and in need of help during 2012. We chatted and discussed what I needed to do to improve my health. It took at least two more years before I was able to really make progress toward improving my health (nutrition and physical activity). The link was that I had completely neglected mind-space because of my workaholic attitude. I had improved my diet and nutrition, but I was still working seventy-hour workweeks, including travel. I finally ran my stress hormone system out of control and experienced a complete "crash-out." I was still basically functional, but nothing was coming easy and the presentations that I gave were no longer crisp. I had finally spread myself too thin.

3) What motivated you to become healthy again? Did you "wake up," or were you always awake but did not act on what you knew you needed to do?

I feel that I was always "aware" about my health, but I had neglected my health due to my career and the poor choices I had made. For example, it's better to not be in a relationship than it is to be in a bad relationship. I am now in a good relationship with support; however, my life had been plagued with draining relationships on both a personal and professional level.

The first thing I realized about my health was that I had food allergies— specifically to wheat, most likely to gluten. With my background in clinical research, I had all the knowledge to recognize what my major food allergies were, but I could not give up breads and other wheat-based foods (specifically beer). I love the different flavors of beer, especially since breweries began springing up everywhere. Most of the time I did not feel fully well because of a wheat sensitivity. This was the first motivation: to get wheat out of my diet. When I made that decision, I weighed 245 pounds. I now weigh 195 pounds.

The second issue I identified was that my spine and central nervous system were a bit out of whack. I was in chronic pain because of a hip and clavicle injury that I had suffered many years before. When I saw Dex, who worked on me to correct my spine, he was incredibly helpful. During this time and treatment, my hip popped in and out of place. This was incredibly painful. After the hip stabilized, the muscle spasm went away after six months! I made the decision that I was going to get back in shape.

My third major issue was just sheer exhaustion from living what I called a "reckless abandon" lifestyle. I am not sure why I was proud of that at the time. It must have been something that I picked up during my life and journey. However, my blood pressure was too high, and I could not concentrate on most things because I was spread across so many projects. I once even passed out from shear stress, breaking my nose, resulting in a terrible concussion. I was not in control; it was time to stop living this lifestyle. Winning is not the only thing in life. Relaxation is also important.

4) Are there specific fad diets/workouts that you tried that didn't work? Did you give up and restart several times, only to go back to being unhealthy?

I generally tried many things that I found not to be useful. I enjoy going to the gym, but it's more fun to go with someone else who also enjoys the gym. Looking back at the data in my journals, it was a full year before I hit a somewhat consistent workout regimen. Prior to that, I had numerous startups that did not stick. The sports injuries that I had over my life also contributed to the lack of consistency. I finally learned that most of my pain comes from sitting at desks for too long with poor form. This was a major contributor to my chronic pain as well.

I tried jogging and treadmills, but I have always disliked long-distance running, which is why I played baseball. I tried swimming, but I sink like a rock for some reason and I don't actually like being in the water. Finally, I discovered cycling, and I found that I really enjoyed it. I think it brings me back to the freedom I had when I was younger, riding my bike everywhere. It offered the freedom to go wherever I wanted.

I never tried a "fad diet." The hardest part of my nutritional goals is keeping the extra added sugar out of my diet. Also, I have to keep wheat-based foods out of my diet. The next time you travel, take a look at the food that is available in an airport, at the cash registers, or just in general with fast food. You might be amazed at what you see when you make this observation. In these cases, the choices are small for those who would like to avoid added sugar and wheat-based products.

5) Did you adopt any new meditative practices, power naps, or prayer schedules that helped "fill your cup" or "ease your mind"?

I am still continuing to work on this particular aspect at times. The practice does not come naturally to me, being a "hyper-creative type." I do find some mental release while cycling, but I consider this more like "Zen". To help ease the mind, I found that meditation works best for me. I practice guided medication with an app called "Mind-Space." I find that this practice helps my years of chronic insomnia. I am a high-strung person at times, so this is hard.

I have also started the practice of "no real thinking or work" when I get up in the morning. I used to wake up and just start going right away. Now, I sit and enjoy my coffee and dogs. Now that I have my morning time, I find that I can manage the daily nuances with improved results. Also, I was always way past my limits with the number of projects and clients that I carried. I have greatly scaled back on sheer volume because it is just not prudent for me to be overloaded. I always thought I was superhuman—and I truly felt superhuman—but in the end, I am just a human. This understanding has allowed my cup to be fuller as I go through my daily routines.

The last piece that I have added is yoga. This has been great for releasing positive energy and has helped my meditative practice.

6) What is your final "N-of-1" regimen for nutrition and physical activity, and how do you maintain the balance (mind-space) you have found? What does your diet now consist of? Do you have a system? (For example, 50% vegetables, 25% meat, 25% carbohydrates, etc.) What are your typical workouts or physical activities for the week? Do you have certain goals that you try to hit during the week?

I call my diet "practical paleo." It's simple: no processed foods or added sugar and because of my food sensitivity, no wheat-based products. I often eat rice and sweet potatoes for my carb source, as well as copious amounts of fruit. I eat leafy vegetables, but I really don't like them. I prefer broccoli, zucchini, etc. over leafy-type veggies. I eat eggs daily and work to get proper "good" fats into my diet.

I say "practical" paleo because I will have cheesecake or other desserts on the weekends. Or, if we go to the movie theater, I get a box of Sour Patch Kids to snack on. Since I have control over what I eat, I can add these desserts and treats to my diet. I would still prefer to have beer, but now I drink wine at social dinners.

Five years ago, I decided to dedicate better practices for my nutrition and physical activity to improve my lifestyle and overall health. First, I started by simply walking a mile. Then two miles. Then three miles. Then I started working out once a week, twice a week, etc., until I built up the momentum to get to where I am today. While working through my workout and building momentum, I also worked to improve my nutrition (gut microbes), and to adopt a practical paleo diet.

Recovery Story 2: Brent F.
Self-Motivation Naturally Leads to a Routine That Works

1) While growing up, what sort of diet did you have, and what sorts of athletic activities did you participate in (high school through college)? Can you describe your diet from that time?

Growing up, I was very athletic and active. I would typically play hours of sports per day, and during my senior year of high school, I joined the cross country and track and field teams. I was very successful in running long distance and earned a track scholarship to Southeastern Louisiana University. Because of my high level of activity, I would eat whatever I wanted. In general, I ate a diverse number of foods (grains, vegetables, fruits, etc.) so, at the time, I thought I had a pretty healthy diet.

2) What were the factors (or reasons) that contributed to your loss in overall health?

After graduating from college, I no longer participated in competitive distance running. For years after, I maintained a decent level of activity (running, weight training). However, I never changed my eating habits. As a result, I began to gain about five pounds a year.

At first, it was no big deal, but at some point, I found myself at 250 pounds. I had become "fat and happy" with two young kids at home, and my focus was on work and them. Occasionally, I would increase my level of exercise to reduce my weight, but it was not very effective. I didn't know how to "diet," so exercise was an easier way for me to try to lose weight. At some point, I reached a breaking point. I believe several factors were involved (increased stress at work, being overweight, and consuming too much alcohol), so I decided that I would change my diet and lose weight.

Unfortunately, how I came to that exact decision is a bit blurry. By changing my diet (with exercise) I lost about fifty pounds in six to eight months. It has been three years, and I am consistently holding 190–195 pounds (down fifty-five to sixty pounds).

3) What motivated you to become healthy again? Did you "wake up," or were you always awake but did not act on what you knew you needed to do?

I slowly became overweight. I really didn't notice it. It snuck up on me. Unfortunately, I do not know what finally triggered my desire to diet and lose weight. Once I figured out that my new diet worked for me to lose weight and I saw a decrease in weight, the competitive athlete in me came out, and it became a "race" between me and my body. I weighed myself almost daily, and when I saw the weight come down, it motivated me even more to keep going. When I slacked off and the weight crept up, I got angry and kicked back into gear. That said, because I stuck to a routine, it really wasn't that hard. These days, the only time I find it hard is on vacations/holidays when sticking to a diet is difficult, but as soon as that time is over, I get right back on my routine and schedule. The key to working out and dieting (for me) was routine. I didn't even think about it. I didn't have to choose to do it. I just did it because that was the routine.

4) Are there specific fad diets/workouts that you tried that didn't work? Did you give up and restart several times, only to go back to being unhealthy?

I have only tried one "diet" in my life, and that is the one that has worked. As a result, I don't call it a diet, I call it a "lifestyle modification."

I don't even know how I came up with this diet. I don't recall reading about it. I do know that I am generally anti-carbs (Americans consume way too much sugar), and I specifically designed my diet to minimize carbs (but I didn't go to extremes like the Atkins diet).

5) Did you adopt any new meditative practices, power naps, or prayer schedules that helped "fill your cup" or "ease your mind"?

I began to do power naps at work, particularly in the early afternoon. I would lie on my office floor with a yoga mat and a small pillow. Not too comfortable, but comfortable enough that I could "zone out" and relax for ten to twenty minutes. At some point, while lying there, I end up wide awake and ready to get up and work again.

6) What is your final N-of-1 regimen for nutrition and physical activity, and how do you maintain the balance (mind-space) you have found? What does your diet now consist of? Do you have a system? (For example, 50% vegetables, 25% meat, 25% carbohydrates, etc.) What are your typical workouts or physical activities for the week? Do you have certain goals that you try to hit during the week?

In my opinion, it is all about finding what works for you. Once you have found something that works for you, it is about making it a part of your new lifestyle and life routine. It is just something you do. If it is something that you "choose" to do every day, then one day, you will decide not to do it anymore, and you'll fall back into old bad habits.

Just like any diet, the key to mine was to lower calorie intake. My diet consisted of a protein shake (made with water, not milk) that I would bring to the office and sip on throughout the day (usually one scoop of protein was adequate for the day). I don't eat breakfast, but if I am at work and I get hungry, I will eat a handful of nuts to hold me over. For lunch, I would eat raw broccoli. At some point, I began to spoil myself and dip the broccoli in a small amount of hummus. I snack on the broccoli throughout the day to keep the hunger at bay. I then eat a normal dinner (whatever I want to eat).

For me, this diet is about three things:

(1) Eating very low carbs throughout the day (not sure if low carbs really matter, or the low calories)

(2) This type of eating has shrunk my stomach, so now I eat less to get the same full feeling

(3) Eating just broccoli makes me slightly nauseous (not enough that I actually feel sick or that it affects my overall health but just enough that it seems to quench my hunger more than eating other foods)

Weekends are a bit harder for me to stay on schedule, so I don't usually follow this routine on the weekends, but I try to be "good." However, when Monday rolls back around, it all starts back up again.

In general, I try to work out six days per week. That might include a run in the morning before work. Or I also try to do weight training two times per week. Occasionally, I will do both in one day (depending on motivation and the amount of time I have).

Recovery Story 3: Jenny G.
Lifestyle Change in Lieu of Medication

1) While growing up, what sort of diet did you have, and what sorts of athletic activities did you participate in (high school through college)? Can you describe your diet from that time?

During my childhood and high school years, we had cereal for breakfast, pasta, meatloaf, potatoes—no real connection with raw foods, just items like green beans and instant potatoes—things that were cheap. During college, I ate whatever I wanted, whenever I wanted. I did not do any athletics in high school or college. I was a lifeguard and swam for fun some during high school.

2) What were the factors (or reasons) that contributed to your loss in overall health?

The factors that contributed to my slip in health were the stress of work, time management, and not knowing how to cook for myself. I did not eat all day and ate fast food all the time. I did not connect my choice of food with my energy level. This caused me to go home and crash. I did not do much activity, I just sat in front of the TV. I did not know that I could be doing more at that time.

3) What motivated you to become healthy again? Did you "wake up," or were you always awake but did not act on what you knew you needed to do?

What woke me up was my knowledge of heart disease being the biggest killer of women and having my own lab work done. After the third time I got my results back, my doctor said that if I didn't change my lifestyle, he would need to put me on medication for cholesterol. At this time, I was sixty pounds overweight. I left his office and went to the gym and hired a trainer because I needed accountability. I did not want to be on that particular medication because of the possible side effects. Based on the knowledge I had, there was no excuse for me to not change my lifestyle; it did take three tests though, through three straight years. It does take time, and I did make sacrifices (don't eat that snack!) It was hard—and it was worth doing. I lost a lot of weight, and I got my cholesterol numbers in proper specs.

4) Are there specific fad diets/workouts that you tried that didn't work? Did you give up and restart several times, only to go back to being unhealthy?

I never really had restrictions on my diet until that day in the doctor's office. Seriously, since I left the doctor's office, I have always worked to maintain a proper diet. It taught me that if I eat fish and vegetables, I could eat more. I connected how I feel with what I eat.

5) Did you adopt any new meditative practices, power naps, or prayer schedules that helped "fill your cup" or "ease your mind"?

I have always liked my morning prayer time, but I started to practice meditation. Now I do both: guided meditation and prayer affirmations. I have recently found that doing both is very helpful to help me maintain balance. It is my normal morning routine.

6) What is your final N-of-1 regimen for nutrition and physical activity, and how do you maintain the balance (mind-space) you have found? What does your diet now consist of? Do you have a system? (For example, 50% vegetables, 25% meat, 25% carbohydrates, etc.)

What are your typical workouts or physical activities for the week? Do you have certain goals that you try to hit during the week?

The typical diet I maintain includes a lot of leafy greens, eggs, coffee— sometimes Bulletproof Coffee (if I do have Bulletproof Coffee, I eat no carbs until at least 2:00 p.m.), a lot of water, a lot of fiber, nuts, dark chocolate, all meats (grass-fed and hormone-free), and bone broth. For my cheats, I like to have things like french fries. Also, I like wine and cheese, of course. For my diet, I found that eliminating dairy, wheat, and low-nutritious carbs has made me feel great!

I go to the gym two to three times per week with a trainer, where I do HITT and weightlifting. I also go to yoga three to six times per month. For cardio and headspace, I try to cycle thirty to sixty miles a week. I have found this to be very therapeutic and fun. It's proper self-care to find activities that you enjoy and to do them regularly. The happier you are, the more likely that you can be the best for everyone else.

I meditate regularly, sometimes guided and sometimes personal. This is the key to clearing my mind for the day. Sometimes, I have to take breaks during the day to remember the sunny sky. It can be really difficult.

Recovery Story 4: Jessica E.
At Age 66, Still Able to Change Her Lifestyle

1) While growing up, what sort of diet did you have, and what sorts of athletic activities did you participate in (high school through college)? Can you describe your diet from that time?

Well, I will generally speak about my life before I made the change two years ago. One of the things I remember from growing up is that we had dessert every night. We baked a pie or had cookies. I think that is why I crave sweets all the time and still do to this day. I did not do this with my kids and made dessert more of a treat. Typically, we were a meat and potatoes family, with salads and bread. We also had pasta all the time. I haven't been "athletic" and wasn't really that "active." Most of my activity was geared toward raising my kids, working, and now helping raise my grandchildren.

2) What were the factors (or reasons) that contributed to your loss in overall health?

I go to the doctor regularly and have never really been in bad health. It really crept up on me over the years. I pushed my health to the edge but never really put myself in "bad" health. During my life, I never overate, I just kept eating what I have always eaten. Over time, our bodies change, and I never really changed anything.

3) What motivated you to become healthy again? Did you "wake up," or were you always awake but did not act on what you knew you needed to do?

Like many people that I hear about, I went to the doctor and received a prediabetic diagnosis. My blood sugar level was at 105. Some of my other numbers were on the edge as well.

The word "prediabetic" scared me. My husband had passed away because of Type 1 diabetes and heart complications. When I received the prediabetic diagnosis, the doctors wanted to start me on a regimen of pills. I did not want to be medicated, so I asked if there were other options. The doctor pointed me to a nutritionist, and since then, I have followed a new diet. Another motivator is that I really want to dance at my grandchildren's weddings. This really motivates me.

4) Are there specific fad diets/workouts that you tried that didn't work? Did you give up and restart several times, only to go back to being unhealthy?

I did try different diets over time, but never a fad diet. However, they did not stick. The diets that didn't work told me to eliminate everything within a particular food type. This was, honestly, too hard because you had to give up everything! When I received the proper nutrition coaching in what I should be eating, as opposed to a diet that stated that I had to stop eating something, my results were much better, and now, I can stick with the diet I have.

5) Did you adopt any new meditative practices, power naps, or prayer schedules that helped "fill your cup" or "ease your mind"?

As we get older, we change, and we can see the finish line. I am the same I have always been—a generally positive person. I have always had a great disposition and mental fortitude. Of course, there are days I am down, but I just talk myself out of it. I really value my own time, even now. I do have a lot of faith and have a personal spiritual connection. In the end, I am pretty realistic about all things within reason and really didn't change anything in that part of my life.

6) What is your final N-of-1 regimen for nutrition and physical activity, and how do you maintain the balance (mind-space) you have found? What does your diet now consist of? Do you have a system? (For example, 50% vegetables, 25% meat, 25% carbohydrates, etc.) What are your typical workouts or physical activities for the week? Do you have certain goals that you try to hit during the week?

For my change in diet, I now eat meat, cheese, and salads. I leave the condiments off my food. I leave off the sauces. It is amazing how many calories come from dressings, sauces, and condiments. For example, all I now use is a dressing of oil, vinegar, salt, and pepper for my salads. I also cut out all of the extra carbs and sugar. For example, we used to have bread at every dinner. Now, we skip that part of the meal. We also don't have dessert that often, either, but I still have treats every once in a while. Since getting my diet under control, I have my cheat days, but I don't overdo it. For example, if I go to dinner, I get a steak, salad, and potatoes. In this case, I will have bread at a restaurant. I don't eat or keep bread at home. Sometimes, I think it's good to have these foods because it resets our systems. If you deprive yourself of everything you love, why bother? It's important to still have some cheat days once in a while so you can live life to its fullest.

For my physical activity, I found that going to the pool every day is fun! I also have a nice tan now. I walk, jog, and work out in the water for about forty-five minutes per day. Also, I have found four or five girlfriends to do this with. It will eventually get too cold to get in the pool, so we will still meet together and start walking around the neighborhood for forty-five minutes. I don't really like exercise, so it has to be fun! We also encourage each other to help maintain our diets and physical activities. This is also a must. Friends encourage me, and I don't want to let anyone down who supports me—even my nutritionist. In the end, we all need someone to help hold us accountable to make it through the cravings and stay on track.

I definitely feel better. Over the last two years since making the change, I have lost sixty-three pounds!

Story 5: Matt C.
How the Desire to See His Children Grow up Changed His Life

1) While growing up, what sort of diet did you have, and what sorts of athletic activities did you participate in (high school through college)? Can you describe your diet from that time?

Growing up, we ate cereal for breakfast, PB&J or ham and cheese sandwiches for lunch, and then pasta and meatballs with salad for dinner. We were really a meat and potatoes family. We also often had lasagna and baked ziti. I did not eat much in the way of veggies growing up, though we did have corn and green beans. For athletic activities, I played baseball and tried a few other sports; however, I had "growing pains" in my knee, as well as childhood asthma. I did enjoy the sports I played and have always liked football. I also tried the weightlifting team and enjoyed it. I was able to work on my upper body without hurting my knees, so this worked for me early in life.

I did not go to college like some of my other friends, but I did start my own company that I sold for some early money. As part of my job, I obtained training in self-defense and was stronger than many of my friends. As I got older, my asthma symptoms went away, but I have always had arthritic knees.

2) What were the factors (or reasons) that contributed to your loss in overall health?

I just did not take care of myself, like most people. I ate whatever I wanted and never really paid attention to where my health was going. I also did not work out and generally did not care to. Especially after leaving high school, I did not have anything organized in my life. My bad eating habits were often related to my job.

I did not really follow any patterns. I had a twenty-four hour, on-call type job and would eat food from the gas station or pick up a hamburger and fries. Single with plenty of money, I always ate out. I also didn't know how to cook, so I was always ordering pizza. If I had all the money back that I spent on pizza in the past twenty-five years, I could probably retire. Until I got married, I did not eat home-cooked meals. This continued into my marriage, and I was just raising my family and going on with life. So, in the end, I was just not paying attention to how I was treating myself. My wife was really patient with me. She is a very loving person and did not question me about my health (too much).

3) What motivated you to become healthy again? Did you "wake up," or were you always awake but did not act on what you knew you needed to do?

My father had diabetes and had heart issues. This has always been on my mind. I knew that I was unhealthy but was content with how I was living my life. I now have three great kids and a loving wife. As I got older, I realized that I probably needed to change my behaviors and habits so I could see my children get older and be successful at what they do.

I had been going to my regular doctor visits, and she told me that I was overweight and needed to start exercising. I wasn't listening. What really changed me was what happened to my brother-in-law. He is ten years older, and we had the same diet—you know, sharing a full plate of brownies. He had a massive heart attack, and it really affected me. I didn't want the same thing to happen to me. I changed my diet and lifestyle because I knew that it would help me possibly live longer to see my kids grow up. Also, my wife is athletic, and I thought it would be fun to start participating in the same events she did.

4) Are there specific fad diets/workouts that you tried that didn't work? Did you give up and restart several times, only to go back to being unhealthy?

I really had the same diet my whole life until I decided to change based on what happened to my brother-in-law. I have never really been into fads in general. I will tell you that the change in my diet has really changed my energy, and I am happy that I have changed. It was an uphill battle because I started this change in my late thirties. I don't normally regret anything from my life, but I wish I would have started earlier because it would have been easier.

5) Did you adopt any new meditative practices, power naps, or prayer schedules that helped "fill your cup" or "ease your mind"?

In short, family time is my time. I enjoy this very much. It is really all I need.

6) What is your final N-of-1 regimen for nutrition and physical activity, and how do you maintain the balance (mind-space) you have found? What does your diet now consist of? Do you have a system? (For example, 50% vegetables, 25% meat, 25% carbohydrates, etc.) What are your typical workouts or physical activities for the week? Do you have certain goals that you try to hit during the week?

The short answer is that I greatly reduced my carbohydrate intake and started going to the gym regularly. I still love my pasta and different Italian meals, but I eat far fewer carbs. I started to eat more vegetables and will not eat any low-value carbs during the week. I also cut out added sugar products and don't eat buns or french fries. I skip dessert most of the time now. Also, I make better choices while out at dinner.

For my physical activity, I really enjoy going to the gym. I go three days per week and have some workout buddies who enjoy it as well. I get my steps in when I can—going to the bus stop, working on things on my property. I look to win the little battles with food and physical activity. It's a fun game. My wife has been competing in the Tough Mudder endurance course for some time. I started doing these competitions with her, and I found it to be incredibly fun. It's fun to be an adult and go play in the mud for some athletic activities. I managed to lose thirty pounds (from 205 to 175) with the changes that I have made. I feel much better and have more energy to keep up with my kids. It seems easy to keep up the diet and exercise because I've noticed that I just generally feel better. It is easy for me to maintain this balance in my mind because I reconnected my nutrition and health to generally feeling better and knowing that I have increased the likelihood that I will live longer.

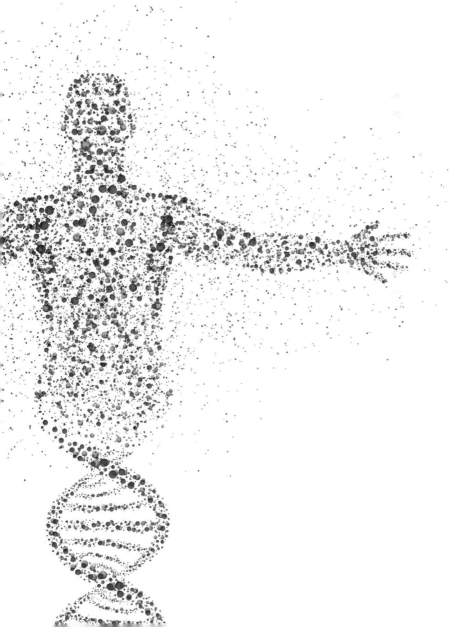

PART 2:

NUTRITION, CARBOHYDRATE CONSUMPTION, DISEASE, AND THE N-OF-1 CHALLENGE

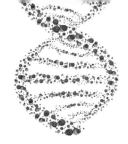

CHAPTER 4:

FOOD CHEMISTRY AND EXCESS CARBOHYDRATES LEADING TO OBESITY

This part of the book is designed to be from the point of view of calorie and carb-counting. My goal is to discuss the different types of carbohydrates and their effect on nutrition and obesity. There are other nutritional aspects that we need to consider for a fully healthy diet besides just calorie and carb-counting; however, if you take the advice in this section, and this book, you may naturally get the nutrients that you need from proper diet changes.

We want to eat meals that come from all food groups. As I mentioned before, one of the main points of this book is to bring awareness to the overuse of food and obesity. One of the goals of Part 2 is to understand something called "Medical Nutritional Therapy" and we want to create personal eating plans and change habits. In the end, you can still enjoy the foods you like, just much less **(REF 5).**

Let's just get this up front and stated: the first thing to do is to drink regular water instead of sugar water **(REF 5, 6).**

"You are what you eat" is the age-old saying. Yet we continue to stuff our faces with excess amounts of food. To start this discussion, I would like to point out that there are certain properties of food that can make it addictive. This has to do with how food interacts with our brain, body, and gut microbiome.

Through my biomedical research activities, travels, and by attending numerous life sciences seminars led by the top experts in biomedical research, I have seen and worked on several types of cutting-edge topics related to health. I would like to share some of the information throughout this part of the book on what I have learned. In the end, I am working to synthesize different relevant topics for easy digestion of information.

When I was working at The Scripps Research Institute in Florida during the middle of the 2000s, my office was down the hall from a professor named Dr. Paul J. Kenny. One of the research topics that he still focuses on is understanding the neurobiological mechanisms of drug addiction, obesity, and schizophrenia. Some of the work that he presented at the seminars included results on food addiction behaviors linked to sugar. He has also published numerous journal articles on his research and has contributed to Scientific America on the topic **(REF 7, 8)**. The articles have a wealth of information and present some of the views on the molecular biology of the food we eat. The results from his research studies, as well as many other experts in the field, revealed that there is a reward pathway in the brain that is linked to sugar and sweets. His study, as well as other researchers, showed that sugar has certain addictive properties and that this addiction works through a similar pathway as other addictive drugs **(REF 7, 8).**

In the article, he states that: "Drugs of abuse, such as morphine, stimulate the brain's reward systems the way food does. Yet the similarities do not end there. When morphine is injected into the striatum of rats, it triggers binges like overeating, even in rats that have been fed to satiety. This response shows that morphine and other opiates mimic the effects of neurotransmitters (brain chemicals) such as endorphins that are naturally produced in the brain to stimulate feeding behaviors" **(REF 7).**

But please understand what I am explaining. Sugar is needed for us to function properly and sugar is definitely needed for brain function. The discussion in my book is more related to what happens when we *overconsume* sugars and complex carbohydrates. I am not calling sugar bad, I am describing how it interacts with our body.

Another research team at The University of California, San Francisco—The SugarScience group—has pulled many studies for review on the topic of food addiction. For example, their website references: "Using brain-scanning technology, scientists at the U.S. National Institute on Drug Abuse were among the first to show that sugar causes changes in peoples' brains similar to those in people addicted to drugs such as cocaine and alcohol. These changes are linked to a heightened craving for more sugar. This important evidence has set off a flood of research on the potentially addictive sugars" **(REF 9).**

Here's a way to look at the conversation on addiction: every time we consume sugar, we get a positive reward in our brain through the dopamine reward pathway. What's interesting is this reward pathway is related to the diets of early humans as we developed into our society today. Refined sugar did not exist for humans prior to the 1500's. Sugar-rich foods were a rare treat, so the reward system was an evolutionary advantage when we were hunter-gathers. This biological pathway was used to reward us for finding sugar: "Good job! You found some sugar. You get a bump of happiness."

Even though we may be weakly addicted to sugar because of our biochemistry, it is nowhere as bad as the addictive properties of opioids or dealing with alcoholism. I don't want to offend anyone that is dealing with these sorts of addictions. However, we want to be aware that there is a chemical aspect while working through a new diet plan. We have powerful minds, and I have seen humans do great things. Anyone who puts consistent effort into any area of his or her life will win. It's the human way. Just like with all types of addiction, the level of sugar addiction is dependent on the individual.

As for a topic that you may not have heard about before, cravings for sugar can be triggered by the microbes that live in our stomachs and guts. Not only do cravings come from our own molecular biology, but the microbes in our gut have been found to be important as well. I will expand on the topic of gut microbes in Chapter 7 of this book.

A nutritional change will take effort, and it may be very difficult to get through a plan. It's like going to the gym; if you only work out once a week, all you are doing is making yourself sore for three days. Without consistency, you can't obtain any benefits. The food that we eat interact with our bodies in similar ways - over the course of multiple days at a time.

At its most basic level, food is just a collection of chemicals. Our bodies digest these chemicals, so we can live. However, over-consumption can make you sick and increase risk factors that can lead to disease. During the next few sections, we are going to review some of the aspects of simple sugars, carbohydrates, calorie counting, and health risk factors for continued overconsumption of food.

A Biochemistry Lesson and Nutrition

The food we eat determines the nutrition that we receive and ultimately determines our health. There are constant chemical reactions going on in our bodies at difficult-to-measure time scales. I say this because it is one of the keys to understanding what is going on in our bodies with regards to the food that we eat. The simple sugar or complex carbohydrates that we eat will simply be used, secreted, or stored. It follows that the biochemistry going on in our bodies is dependent on how much we eat, when we eat, and what we eat. Thus, nutrition is essentially controlled by chemistry and the biological systems that help convert food into molecules that our bodies need to survive. But let's just focus on simple sugars and complex carbohydrates.

If you are consuming more sugar and carbohydrates than you can use for energy, your body will start to store the food for future use. If not stored or used, the food gets secreted. So, it is simple logic that if you continue to consume excess amounts of carbohydrates, you will gain weight because it will be stored around your belly and other parts of your body. If you never use the fat that is stored, because you are not active, then how are you going to lose weight? We are what we eat.

The terms sugar, carbohydrates, lipids, and fats can have different meanings based on who you ask. We hear about them all the time, but how many people know what their chemical structures look like? These classes of molecules are often spoken of in vague terms for what they are and what they do for us. It can be easy to forget that these terms represent real, physical molecules that interact with our bodies to produce life. With my background in clinical research and biochemistry, I often think in terms of chemical structure, metabolism/catabolism rate, biochemical pathway, etc.

Below and on the next page, I have included some chemical structures that are common in everyday use. Even if you don't have a background in chemistry or biochemistry, the point is to pay attention to the structure of the molecule and to simply consider that the structure dictates how it is used by our bodies. For fun, see if you can name the molecules in the figure. The purpose of this exercise is to try to assign the molecule to what we are consuming and its effects.

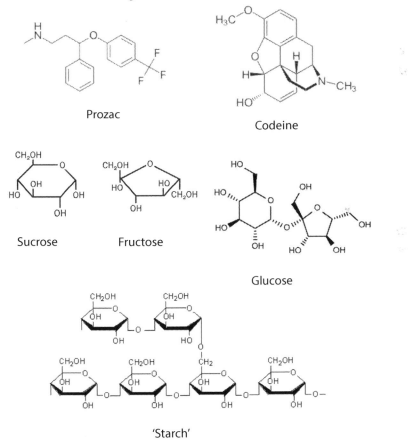

Figure 1a – Chemical structures of common molecules found in everyday life.

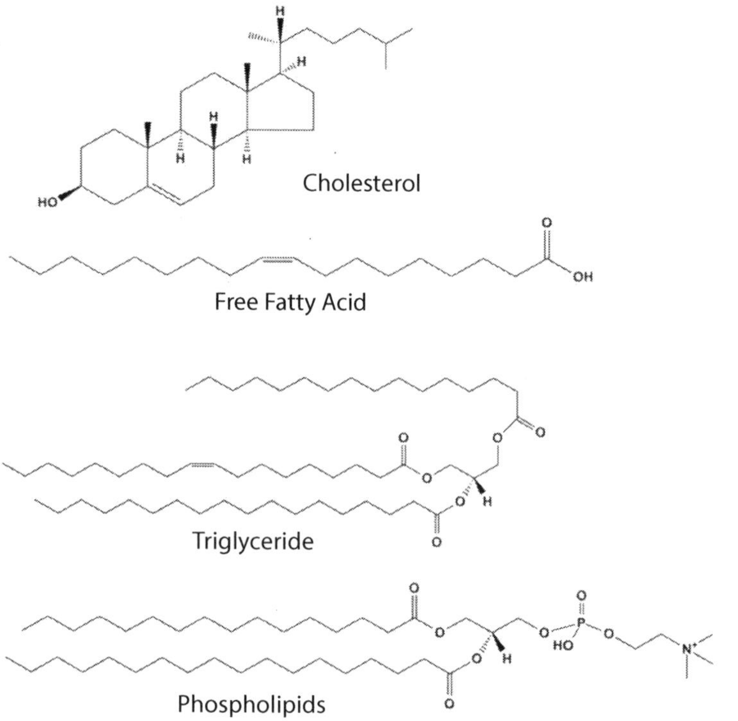

Figure 1b - Chemical structures of common molecules found in everyday life.

The first two molecules at the top of **Figure 1a** are Prozac and Codeine. I started with these molecules because the names are common in our society. Most people are aware of what Prozac and Codeine are and what they do. Prozac is used to treat ADHD in children, and Codeine is overprescribed and used for pain. Think about it, these molecules interact with our bodies to create changes and physiological effects. For example, Prozac creates a sense of calm, and Codeine suppresses pain. Next, let's think about sugar and carbohydrates. In the same sense, think about how they interact with our bodies.

The next molecules are sucrose, fructose, and glucose in the second row of **Figure 1a**. This is what is often referred to as sugar. Note, these are relatively small molecules. The last molecule in **Figure 1a** is general starch—a chain of sugars making a much larger molecule. This is considered a complex carbohydrate. We will expand the discussion on sugar and carbohydrates later during this chapter.

Figure 1b shows cholesterol, a free fatty acid, and lipids. Often, we speak about cholesterol in terms of the levels in our blood, as well as good and bad cholesterol. The topic of cholesterol is within itself another topic of discussion that is associated with obesity. Problems with cholesterol can be associated with many other steroids and hormones in our bodies, but in the end, we can measure this class of molecules. Analytical chemists and biochemists design tests to measure cholesterol so that we can use them as health markers. We have and can design all sorts of tests to measure these different molecules of importance.

The other molecules shown are types of lipids. Molecules such as free fatty acids, triglycerides, and phospholipids are important for regulating obesity and general well-being. These lipid molecules are generally considered to be fats, which is also important to consider when pursuing nutritional changes. Wherever you are with your health and when developing your personal diet plan, calories from fats should also be considered. However, there is currently a wide debate regarding good fats versus bad fats and diets. I personally believe that we are "good fat" deprived in this country and that we should reduce the amount of sugar that we consume to help avoid obesity. I believe that overconsumption of sugar and carbohydrates is the major contributing factor to obesity. As we go through the chapter, you will see why I am focusing on sugar and carbohydrates.

We could get quite detailed on the field of nutrition, but I'm going to keep it fairly narrow in this book. I am discussing the benefits of:

- Reducing or eliminating excess or refined sugar consumption
- Reducing excess carbohydrate consumption
- Reducing meal portions
- Generally reducing food with high calorie counts

Simple Carbohydrates

Commonly, carbohydrates can be classified into two subsets: simple or complex. Simple carbohydrates include sugars such as glucose, fructose, and sucrose (Review **Figure 1a** again for structures.) These types of carbohydrates are used quickly because they are primed for use. Note that they are physically smaller than a starch; i.e. the complex starch will take more time for our bodies to break down.

Sugar is needed for brain function, but when you consume copious amounts of sugar in a day, without really performing physical activity, what do you think will happen? The body will most likely start to store the extra carbohydrates. I think that it is commonly known that there are many sources of sugars, as well as artificial sweeteners. Some of these include:

- High-fructose corn syrup (mostly fructose, not glucose)
- Artificial sweeteners (aspartame, sucralose, and saccharin)
- Sugar alcohols (sorbitol, xylitol, mannitol)
- Natural sweeteners (honey, agave, maple syrup, dates, stevia, and fruit)

I suggest that you go to the internet and look at the information on the different types of artificial sweeteners. Is "diet soda" *really* designed for you to lose weight? Or is it meant to be an "alternative diet" to added-sucrose drinks?

With labels, make sure that you understand what the word "diet" means. A diet is defined as what you eat; it does not technically imply any degree of inherent health or nutrition.

For sugar, I personally try to use natural sweeteners. I work to stay away from high fructose syrup, artificial sweeteners, or sugar alcohols. There are sources of sugar that are better than others. For example, dark chocolate (70% cocoa) provides good prebiotics which promote gut health while also providing sugar and other anti-inflammatories. This does *not*, however, mean you should eat a candy bar every day, just that it is a better choice.

Complex Carbohydrates

Complex carbohydrates have molecular structures with complex sugar chains (Review **Figure 1a**). It takes time for the body to break down these chains and convert the molecules into the simple sugars. Complex carbohydrate-type foods often come with minerals, vitamins, and fiber (but not all). Since it takes more time to digest these complex carbohydrates, the increase in simple sugar in the blood occurs at a slower rate.

There are, of course, better choices between different types of carbohydrates. This is because some foods will be digested faster or slower than others. Here's a way to look at it: some foods will dump sugar into the blood at a faster rate. An example of this is white potatoes and processed bread, which contain mostly starch. They have little fiber, and they often lack other nutrients. They can be digested faster than other types of carbohydrates. This is especially important for those that are obese, have prediabetes, or generally have high blood sugar.

To help understand the different types of complex carbohydrate foods and how they directly affect blood sugar level, researchers developed what is call the "glycemic index." One of the reasons that the glycemic index was developed was to aid medical doctors that are treating patients with prediabetes and Type 2 diabetes. The guide is also good for those of us trying to lose weight or wanting to maintain a healthy diet. You can also start now to avoid an obesity-related disease. The effect of consuming simple sugars and the direct increase of the amount in the bloodstream is easily measured and understood; it is literally the number of sugar molecules per volume of blood. Since complex carbohydrates must be digested before they can be used for energy or other processes, the glycemic index is helpful for describing all sorts of food and the effect on blood sugar levels.

Glycemic Index

The glycemic index is a scale that measures how quickly carbohydrates are digested before sugar is released into the blood. The index values also consider if there are other nutrients or fiber that help promote positive health influences. The scale goes from 0 to 100, and with increasing value, describes how quickly a type of food will raise the blood glucose levels. The purpose of this section is to gain awareness about the foods we eat and how they affect the blood sugar levels, or how quickly they may be used. Another way to think about this -Will the extra carbohydrates just be stored in reserves because we are not performing any physical activity? For a reference, Harvard Medical School (HMS) has published a glycemic index for over sixty foods **(REF 10, 11, 12)**. An example of some of the values for the glycemic index can be found in the table below (**Table 1**).

FOOD	Glycemic index (glucose = 100)
HIGH-CARBOHYDRATE FOODS	
White wheat bread*	75 ± 2
Whole wheat/whole meal bread	74 ± 2
Specialty grain bread	53 ± 2
BREAKFAST CEREALS	
Cornflakes	81 ± 6
Wheat flake biscuits	69 ± 2
Porridge, rolled oats	55 ± 2

FOOD	Glycemic index (glucose = 100)
FRUIT AND FRUIT PRODUCTS	
Apple, raw†	36 ± 2
Orange, raw†	43 ± 3
Banana, raw†	51 ± 3
VEGETABLES	
Potato, boiled	78 ± 4
Potato, instant mash	87 ± 3
Carrots, boiled	39 ± 4

Table 1 - HMS Glycemic Index - Partial List

The HMS guidance has recommended the following interpretations of the values: Food types that have a rating of less than 55 are considered low glycemic foods. A rating of greater than 70 is considered a high-glycemic food. Of course, we have the medium-range glycemic foods that fall between 55 and 70. A full list for your review can be found on the HMS webpage **(REF 10)**, as well as other sources not refenced.

To start, let's discuss overeating and processed white bread. If you eat copious amounts of bread every night, this is the first place to look for empty carbohydrates. Processed white bread has a glycemic index of 75 +/- 2 (note: glucose = 100). Whole oats, meanwhile, have a glycemic index of 55 +/- 2. The simple interpretation: If you swap bread with oats and consume the *same* number of calories, the oats will release energy for longer periods throughout the day than the bread. The sugar gets released into the blood faster after eating the bread. If you have a slow release during the day, you can be fueled without the spike in sugar expected from a candy bar or from processed wheat products. One thing that I did early during my N-of-1 Challenge was to eliminate sugar from my coffee. There all sorts of different sources of sugar that we consume each day. We just don't notice because they are habits that we don't admit that we have.

Another important aspect of one's diet is fiber. High-fiber foods are low on the glycemic index because there are fewer complex carbohydrates to break down. Your body will be healthy if you chose foods that contain high fiber. Another trend in the U.S. is that we do not have enough fiber in our diets. Since the advent of the glycemic index, researchers have developed something called the "glycemic load." However, the glycemic load follows the same logic as the glycemic index. The glycemic load has higher importance on the number of carbohydrates found in the food. The scale is similar to the glycemic index and foods found on the high and low scale are essentially the same. A glycemic load of 20 or more is high, and a score of 10 or under is low. Of course, the logic follows that food low on the glycemic load scale is healthy for those of us that need to lose a few extra pounds to avoid obesity-related disease **(REF 10, 11, 12)**.

The following lists are from the Harvard T.H. Chan School of Public Health – The Nutrition Source **(REF 11, 12)**.

Low glycemic load (10 or under)
- Bran cereals
- Apple
- Orange
- Kidney beans
- Black beans
- Lentils
- Cashews
- Nuts
- Carrots

Medium glycemic load (11-19)
- Pearled barley: 1 cup cooked
- Brown rice: 3/4 cup cooked
- Oatmeal: 1 cup cooked
- Bulgur: 3/4 cup cooked
- Rice cakes: 3 cakes
- Whole grain bread: 1 slice
- Whole-grain pasta: 1 1/4 cup cooked

High glycemic load (20+)
- Baked potato
- French fries
- Refined breakfast cereal: 1 oz
- Sugar-sweetened beverages: 12 oz
- Candy bars: one 2-oz bar or three mini bars
- Couscous: 1 cup cooked
- White basmati rice: 1 cup cooked
- White-flour pasta: 1 1/4 cup cooked (15)"

Several studies have shown an association between consuming high glycemic-index foods with an increase in risk for obesity, prediabetes, or Type 2 diabetes, and heart disease. It follows that foods low on the glycemic index have shown to help with weight loss and to help control Type 2 diabetes. For the N-of-1 Challenge, I suggest replacing some of your high-glycemic foods with more nutritious, lower-glycemic foods.

Following the principles of low-glycemic eating can be a guide for choosing food. The overall goal is to reach and stay at a healthy weight, so you do not increase risk factors for other diseases. For more information on specific foods, please see information in the HMS or CDC websites **(REF 5, 6)**. Please remember, resources like the glycemic index and load by HMS are just tools that help us make decisions. They help us drive our own N-of-1 Challenge goals.

Overall, the lower on the glycemic index your foods are, the more likely you will be to achieve weight loss. People who are healthier and perform cardio workouts or power lift will need food to complement their diet for the needed energy, i.e. food higher on the index. In a vacuum, if I were to present this conversation to a powerlifter, where the goal is to add weight and muscle, I would rightfully be told I was wrong about my diet suggestion to this group. Remember - this discussion is about what to do if we want to lose extra pounds or if we have let our health slip.

Now that we've had a quick discussion on what sugar and carbohydrates are and have discussed the biochemistry of food, the next step is to start counting the calories we are consuming. The glycemic index and glycemic load are tools that allow us to understand how food interacts with our bodies. In the next chapter, I will present some more tools to help with weight loss, including what is called the body mass index (BMI) and calorie counting.

Seeing a calorie calculation can definitely help us understand how much we are overconsuming food, particularly carbohydrates. It is simple math and can be very eye- opening. This is where I started my journey and N-of-1 Challenge to lose my extra fifty-five pounds—I simply started calorie counting. I love data and analyzing it; you really can't argue with solid data. We also introduce the concept of journaling in the next chapter.

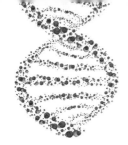

CHAPTER 5:

NUTRITION, THE BODY MASS INDEX, CALORIE COUNTING AND OVER-CONSUMPTION OF REFINED SUGAR

When I realized that I was consuming two times more calories than I needed in a week, it was easy to see that I needed to eat less. I was receiving about 75% of my carbs from sugar and carbohydrates. While changes in my diet took hold during a three-year period, I lost 65 pounds, bringing me back to my sophomore college weight of 185 pounds. At 185 pounds, I was not healthy again—I was ten pounds underweight! In the end, the healthy weight that I should live is between 192 to 198 pounds. Thus, I added the proper muscle weight to get back to 195 pounds -it's hard work to stay at a certain weight all the time. Forming habits to maintain a certain lifestyle can take time. It took three years to reach what I consider my optimal health.

At 195 pounds, I am at my optimal Body Mass Index value (BMI) for the level of activity that I perform. The BMI is a common calculation used to define obesity based on one's height, weight, and percentage of body fat. BMI can be calculated with a simple equation; if you want to perform a quick BMI calculation, Google "BMI calculator." Also, if you visit your doctor or even your local gym, you can probably get a more precise measurement of your BMI or your percentage of body fat.

To help understand BMI and its usage, The National Institute of Health (NIH) has set some guidelines for BMI calculations, as well as additional information **(REF 13)**:

"BMI is a useful measure of overweight and obesity. It is calculated from your height and weight. BMI is an estimate of body fat and a good gauge of your risk for diseases that can occur with more body fat. The higher your BMI, the higher your risk for certain diseases such as heart disease, high blood pressure, Type 2 diabetes, gallstones, breathing problems, and certain cancers" **(REF 13)**.

General BMI Numbers

Underweight	Below 18.5
Normal	18.5–24.9
Overweight	25.0–29.9
Obesity	30.0 and Above

This information can also be found on the Center for Disease Control and Prevention About Adult BMI webpage **(REF 14)**. An expanded discussion is also found on this webpage.

Keep in mind that BMI is another *tool* used to describe risk factors. For our discussion, if you have a BMI higher than 25, you should get a more precise measurement of your percentage body fat to find out what your true optimal weight should be. If your BMI is above 25, we recommend that you visit your doctor for an assessment. If you have a BMI above 30, you should consider taking your doctor's advice. If you have not been to a doctor or specialist in several years, now might be a good time to visit. Don't let your BMI value continue to creep up; this means not only a bigger waistline but an increased risk for diseases linked to obesity. Obesity is a chronic condition that gets worse over time. It does not happen overnight.

A third resource for BMI information includes the National Institute of Diabetes and Digestive and Kidney Diseases Health Information Center **(REF 15)**. The information above for the BMI is a general guideline for BMI considerations. Research has found that optimal BMI can also be linked to national demographics and heritage. The following table expands on the above guidelines for BMI values.

Non Asian American or Pacific Islander		Asian American		Pacific Islander	
At-risk BMI ≥ 25		At-risk BMI ≥ 23		At-risk BMI ≥ 26	
Height	Weight	Height	Weight	Height	Weight
4'10"	119	4'10"	110	4'10"	124
4'11"	124	4'11"	114	4'11"	128
5'0"	128	5'0"	118	5'0"	133
5'1"	132	5'1"	122	5'1"	137
5'2"	136	5'2"	126	5'2"	142
5'3"	141	5'3"	130	5'3"	146
5'4"	145	5'4"	134	5'4"	151
5'5"	150	5'5"	138	5'5"	156
5'6"	155	5'6"	142	5'6"	161
5'7"	159	5'7"	146	5'7"	166
5'8"	164	5'8"	151	5'8"	171
5'9"	169	5'9"	155	5'9"	176
5'10"	174	5'10"	160	5'10"	181
5'11"	179	5'11"	165	5'11"	186
6'0"	184	6'0"	169	6'0"	191
6'1"	189	6'1"	174	6'1"	197
6'2"	194	6'2"	179	6'2"	202
6'3"	200	6'3"	184	6'3"	208
6'4"	205	6'4"	189	6'4"	213

Table 2. Expanded BMI Table for Heritage and Demographics

Table 2 presents the expanded view of BMI, including heritage and demographics. I live at the high end of my BMI (highlighted in grey), but when you replace fat with muscle, your percentage of body fat is lower. In my opinion, the BMI does lack a normalization for the percentage of body fat, but this is not an excuse to ignore the value—especially if you are not physically active. If you are not physically active, and in the 25 to 30 BMI range, the percentage of body fat becomes a valuable piece of information as well.

Awareness is **Step 1**. Let's say your BMI is 34. Okay. So, what now? What sort of diet should you pursue? Should you get a coach or a nutrition expert? Is there someone you can ask for advice on what you should change?

Step 2 is to start recording what you are eating and work to change your diet. Evaluate and change your diet as needed.

Fads and Long-Term Diets

I would like to make a distinction between a fad and a long-term diet. A long-term diet is one where you plan and choose to eat healthy food and not to overconsume loaded sugar drinks, low-value carbs, etc. There are many fad diets that I will not give free advertisement to. If you are being sold short-term diet results, you are probably going to get short-term results. A long-term diet will initially be difficult to enable, but it is manageable.

Once you build momentum with your own N-of-1 Challenge, you can practice what is called an elimination-addition diet to see what makes you feel good or bad. We can even call it a substitution diet. For example, start exchanging out carbohydrate sources that are high on the glycemic index with foods that are lower on the scale. If you eat pasta, switch over to rice for a few weeks to see how you feel with that particular change. Or, if you add sugar to your coffee every day, don't add the sugar and only add the milk or the cream. The goal of this diet plan should be to stop consuming copious amounts of loaded sugar drinks and low-value carbohydrate sources, all the time.

This doesn't mean that you can't have pizza, cake, or a soda every once in a while. It means that you should not have pizza and sugary soda every day of the week. That said, while working toward your N-of-1 Challenge goals, you may want to consider completely eliminating pizza, cake, and soda from your diet initially—to be brought back at a later time.

For more information on an elimination-addition diet, please see my website for some help on how to plan this type of diet. (www.nof1challenge.com). There are different philosophies on this type of diet plan. One camp says that we should be working on eliminating food, while another camp discusses that we should be changing diet by addition. I find that it's best to follow both philosophies at first. I like the word substitution. Often, people get caught up in jargon instead of paying attention to what the message actually is. Like I said before, try to eliminate bread from your diet, but substitute it by eating rice or oats (elimination-addition). Eliminate or reduce the amount of processed sugar from your diet, but then consider adding fruit for sugar.

Counting Calories from Sugar and Carbohydrates

A calorie is defined as a unit of heat energy—hence the term, "burning" calories while we workout. To start this conversation, please look at **Table 3** for the "recommended daily caloric intake" amounts by age and activity level **(REF 16)**. In the following section, I will base all of my calorie-counting calculations on this table as a reference point.

Age	Men			Women		
	Sedentary	Medium	Active	Sedentary	Medium	Active
21-25	2,400	2,800	3,000	2,000	2,200	2,400
26-30	2,400	2,600	3,000	1,800	2,200	2,400
31-35	2,400	2,600	3,000	1,800	2,000	2,200
36-40	2,400	2,600	2,800	1,800	2,000	2,200
41-45	2,200	2,600	2,800	1,800	2,000	2,200
46-50	2,200	2,400	2,800	1,800	2,000	2,200
51-55	2,200	2,400	2,800	1,600	1,800	2,200
56-60	2,200	2,400	2,600	1,600	1,800	2,200
61-65	2,200	2,200	2,600	1,600	1,800	2,000
66-70	2,200	2,200	2,600	1,600	1,800	2,000
71-75	2,200	2,200	2,600	1,600	1,800	2,000

Table 3 – Age, activity level, and general caloric needs

Based on this table, if you are a male in your 40's, the calculated number of calories you need during a year will be 800,800 (2,200 calories x 7 days x 52 weeks). A male in their twenties need 873,600 calories per year. The simple calculation is that you need 72,800 fewer calories per year in your forties than your twenties.

Please note that most of these recommendations are not for endurance athletes or those that are bodybuilding. The recommendations in this book are more about using a carbohydrate-restricted diet to help burn fat to reduce obesity and lose weight. Meals should still be balanced, which is why I suggested the elimination-addition diet. The goal of weight loss is different than the goals of endurance training or for bodybuilders.

To start off with something that we all may already know, consuming numerous sugar drinks in a day or week is generally unhealthy. To continue the counting exercise, let's look at the number of calories in a typical soda drink.

12 oz (355 ml) Can of Soda

Sugars, total:	39g
Calories, total:	140
Calories from sugar:	140

20 oz (590 ml) Bottle of Soda

Sugars, total:	65g
Calories, total:	240
Calories from sugar:	240

1 Liter (34 oz) Bottle of Soda

Sugars, total:	108g
Calories, total:	400
Calories from sugar:	400

Originally, these drinks were designed to be a source of relief after a long day's work—work that included *physical labor.* They were designed to be drunk during the middle of the workday during a break. They were not, however, designed to be consumed while sitting at a desk all day, performing little to no physical activity.

Based on these numbers above, drinking 3 or 4 cans of soda during a day comes to 720 to 960 calories. Over a week, that would be 5,040 to 6,720 calories per week. Now, let's add six to eight beers on the weekend. (A typical beer is between 110 and 200 calories, so let's take the median at 155 calories for the calculation.)

7 beers x 155 calories = 1,055 calories

The soda and beer products alone in this dietary regimen add up to about 7,255 calories consumed in liquid form every week. A look back at **Table 3** will show that 7, 255 calories is about 3 1/2 days of necessary caloric intake, or about 50% (7,255 / 15,400).

This simple exercise for looking at the number of calories that we consume is very important. Calorie counting is one of the best tools we have for helping us understand overuse and food consumption.

How Much Sugar Is Too Much? Recommendations and More Calorie Calculations

Here are some guidelines from the American Heart Association as to what we should actually be consuming with regards to raw, refined sugar **(REF 17)**.

The American Heart Association (AHA) recommended the upper limits of added sugar intake to be 100 calories (6 teaspoons) per day. The calculations for a full year would be:

> 25 grams x 4 = 100 calories
>
> 100 calories x 365 days
>
> = 36,400 calories per year (9,100 grams)
>
> = 20 pounds per year

In other words, the AHA recommends 20 pounds per year of consumption for "added sugar" type food. The World Health Organization (WHO) website says that we should have no more than 30 grams per day (24 pounds per year) of added sugar and that our total calorie count should be less than 5% of our required calories **(REF 18)**.

To continue looking at the numbers, in 2009 it was estimated that 50% of Americans consumed upwards of 170 pounds a year in sugar alone, but what's truly disturbing is that this stat does not include other carb sources. This is just sugar. Let's look at the numbers for the high end of sugar consumption.

> 150 pounds of sugar = 68,039 grams
>
> 1 gram of sugar = 4 calories
>
> Total calories from sugar over one year at 150 pounds
>
> = 272,156 calories

Now, let's consider a year's worth of calories needed for a male at age forty who practices a low amount of physical activity.

> 2,200 calories per day x 365 days = 800,800 calories
>
> 272,156 calories of added sugar @ 150 pounds per year
>
> divided by 800,800 recommended caloric intake per year
>
> @ 40 years old and not active
>
> = ~34% of total needed caloric intake

That means that sugar consumption alone makes up more than one-third of the yearly carb allowance if you consume 150 pounds of sugar each year. Things get even more alarming when we add bread ("Wheat Calories") to the equation. There are about 2,000 calories in a loaf of white bread. What if we average two loaves a week at 2,000 calories?

> 2,000 calories x 2 loafs of bread a week = 4,000
> 4,000 x 52 weeks = 208,000 calories per year
> 208,000 calories / 800,800 (recommended caloric intake)
> = 26%

This is about one-fourth of your recommended yearly carbs. Thus, 150 pounds of refined sugar a year with two loafs of processed white bread per week can make up roughly 60% to 70% of your total yearly calories, before considering the other food you eat!

When we think about the term empty carbs, this is the case we should think about. There are so many other great sources of carbohydrates that don't include sugar drinks or other foods that are high on the glycemic index. I sought to *eliminate* empty carbs, i.e. foods lacking nutrients the body needs. I chose to *add* different types of foods that had nutrients and complex carbohydrates. I rapidly lost weight when I made this choice.

One quick thought: calorie counting doesn't take into effect what your glucose blood concentration will be after consuming those sodas or beer. As we described in the glycemic index portion of this chapter, this refers to the amount of sugar per volume of blood flowing through your body. Also, calorie counting does not consider other nutrients that may be in the food. This is why we have a tool like the glycemic index—to help understand what foods are good for the slow release of sugar into the bloodstream.

Over-Producing and Over-Consuming Sugar – How Did We Get Here as a Society?

Sugar, at one point in history, was a luxury item not freely available to everyone. A large gut was a thing for the wealthy; it was a sign of their wealth. Refined sugar was a very small part of the diet of the other 99.5% of the world's population. Most sugar sources before the 1700s were from pulses, fruits, and vegetables. Also, Before the 1700s, sugar was similar in value to items such as pearls, musk, and spices from India **(REF 19)**.

But when the new world was discovered, the powers of Europe found new commodities to grow, trade, and sell. The Portuguese first learned that the soil and climate in Brazil were primed to grow copious amounts of sugarcane. They introduced the crop to North America and the Caribbean and the Sugar "gold rush" was started **(REF 19)**. The British Royal Navy continued this trend while growing into a world power. The discovery of fertile land helped to power the newly developed empire. As well, more European countries got into the commodities game—the French, the Dutch, and the Spanish- they too started producing tons of sugar. Very quickly, sugar grew to represent 90% of all exports from some of the Caribbean islands, and the world began to consume more processed sugar. Currently, sugar cane is the third most valuable crop in the world **(REF 19)**.

The increase in sugar production dropped the price, making it affordable for most people in Europe to purchase. This increase in added sugar changed the everyday diets of humans living in Europe and the world in general. We started to add sugar to everything. The average western European was consuming about four pounds per year during 1700. Take a look at how that changed **(REF 20, 21)**.

> 1700 – 4 pounds
> 1800 – 22 pounds
> 1850 – 36 pounds
> 1900 – 90 pounds

In an attempt to graph sugar consumption over the years, a document prepared by Stephan Guyenet and Jeremy Laden extracted data from 184 years of per-capita sales of sugar from 1822 to 2005 **(REF 22, 23)**. The date they presented was obtained from the U.S. Department of Commerce and Labor Department, and the U.S. Department of Agriculture (USDA).

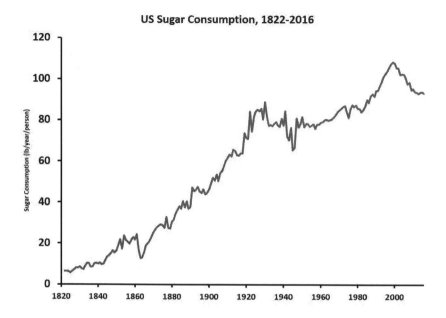

Figure 2 - U.S. Sugar Consumption/Sales during a 184-year period. Data adapted with permission from Author.

One factor that should be considered is that this graph is based on sugar sales, not sugar consumption. Certain assumptions can be made for consumption data based on the per-capita sales of sugar. For this data set, they assumed a 28.8% loss between sales and consumption. The dips in sugar consumption in the chart were mostly dependent on war-time events. For example, there was a reduction in the amount of sugar consumed during WWI and WWII because of rations and money being put towards the war efforts **(REF 22, 23)**. If you do look at this reference, it is called, "By 2606, the U.S. Diet will be 100 Percent Sugar" **(REF 23)**. I don't agree with the extrapolation of this data to that end. However, outside of that extrapolation, the authors did pool excellent data together to illustrate how the consumption of sugar has greatly increased over the last several hundred years.

When looking at multiple sources of data related to, pounds of sugar consumed by the population per year, there are some differences on the exact values. However, if we look at the general trends, we now consume much more refined sugar than we did during the beginning of the 1900's. Now, let's take a deeper look at the data. Right now, we are looking at the "big-data" properties of the information. Remember the conversation on "big-data" during the first part of this book?

Some data indicates that 50% of Americans consume over 110 to 160 pounds of sugar each year. A quick explanation of that data: Let's assume that 50% of Americans consume on average 50 pounds a year and 50% consume 150 pounds. That makes the overall average about 100 pounds. Because we are "averaging" the amount of sugar we consume in a year, we don't see the top-end consumption, 175 pounds, versus those on the low end, around 40 pounds. This is what I mean when I say that we cannot use big-data to see certain problems. It is easy to misuse information and statistics to mask real trends. However, it is easy to see—based on all of the data—that there has been a 2 to 7 times increase in the average amount of sugar being consumed per capita. Regardless of the exact values, we are consuming copious amounts of refined, added sugar.

The data is obvious. Society has changed with respect to nutrition based on sugar production. When sugar started being mass-produced, it was transformed from a luxury item to a commodity, and everyone started to consume more and more, bringing us to today's dilemma with health. At some point, the increase in sugar consumption helped society. But we became greedy and went way past what our limits should be for production and consumption. Think about what we could do with all of that land that currently grows sugar cane.

So, in the end, some of the problems with over-consumption of refined sugar can be related to the overproduction of sugar.

I hope that I have built a picture that allows you to understand that willpower is not necessarily the full problem with obesity. This is why habit formation is so important. Without changing habits, we will not be able to manage our food consumption, and thus not be able to manage obesity. In the next chapter, I will cover information on obesity and the risk factors associated with this trend.

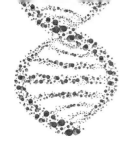

CHAPTER 6:

OBESITY AS A RISK FACTOR FOR DISEASE (PREDIABETES AND TYPE 2 DIABETES)

I would like to start off with a quotation from "Sugar Rush! How Sugar Consumption is Changing America," by Avail Clinical Research on the topics of sugar and diabetes. "It is a myth that eating too much sugar is a direct cause of diabetes. While sugar may not be the direct cause, a diet that is high in sugar can lead to obesity, which in turn can lead to increased risk of diabetes." **(REF 24)**

One of the major crises we are currently experiencing as a society is a growing population of prediabetic and Type 2 diabetes diagnosis—and more so in certain populations. Here are some of the statistics for diabetes diagnosis during 2015 **(REF 25, 26)**.

- 9.4% of the U.S. population has diabetes - 30,300,000+
- Diabetes is the 7th leading cause of death in the U.S.; diabetes is listed as a contributor to 252,806+ deaths per year
- 35.7% of adults are obese (100,000,000+ cases)

Type 2 diabetes represents 90% of all diabetes cases, meaning that only about 10% of diabetes cases are Type 1. Plus, the numbers above only represent confirmed diagnoses of diabetes. To further illustrate the severity of this epidemic, the CDC estimates that one in three Americans is prediabetic: about 84.1 million people. Here are some numbers to understand what 84 million people really means:

- Total U.S. population in 2017: 325.7 million people
- Total population of NY-NJ-PA metro area: 20.3 million residents
- Total population of the state of Florida: 21 million
- Population of Germany: 83 million

These numbers are staggering to contemplate, but awareness is the first step. According to the National Health and Nutrition Examination Survey in 2014, more than 2 in 3 American adults was overweight, and 1 in 13 was obese **(REF 26)**. These were quick numbers on the disease, but now let's answer a question. What exactly is diabetes?

What Is Diabetes?

"Diabetes is a disease of metabolism, which is the way the body uses food for energy. It is related to food nutrients that supply energy called carbohydrates. To move glucose out of blood and into the cells, the pancreas makes a hormone called insulin" **(REF 27)**.

Simply stated, if the cells can't make enough insulin, they cannot use glucose the way that they should. Glucose builds up in the blood, causing diabetes. This means that we would have high blood sugar. To be honest, the disease is still not fully understood, but there are multiple factors that we know contribute to the onset of the disease. Obesity is one of the major factors for developing diabetes. This is because obesity reduces the body's ability to control blood sugar; it is just too much stress on the pancreas to handle this situation **(REF 27)**. This is why I have chosen to discuss only carbohydrates, refined sugar, and the number of calories that we consume each day.

Insulin is a hormone that is synthesized in the pancreas that allows our bodies to use the sugar (glucose) from carbohydrates, as well as helping with the fat storage mechanism. If you have more sugar in your bloodstream, you need more insulin. Thus, Type 2 diabetes develops when the muscles and other cells in our bodies stop responding to insulin, creating a medical condition called insulin resistance. The body can no longer use insulin properly.

However, the body is designed to go into "overdrive" for the sugar-insulin system, but there is a finite amount of insulin that can be produced over time. This means that sugar and insulin biological systems can become saturated. Over time, the glucose in the blood rise because we cannot create enough insulin. In my opinion, after years of abuse, we can "burn out" or "over-use" pancreatic production of insulin, thus the sugar cannot be used and the blood glucose levels spike. The effects of insulin resistance cause sugar levels to maintain high concentrations in the blood. Because of the heavy load on the cells that make insulin, they eventually stop producing it altogether. This process is normally associated with years of poor nutrition habits and is not always associated with genetics **(REF 28)**.

Insulin also affects a hormone name leptin, a natural appetite suppressant that is activated to tell your body that you are not hungry. It's interesting to note: in the biochemical pathways associated with sugar metabolism, we can also have a condition called leptin resistance. When this happens, the body's hunger mechanism is not turned off. We think that we are hungry, keep eating, and start to put the pounds on. This biological system of hunger can work to our disadvantage, given that most of us are able to get our hands-on food anytime we want **(REF 29)**.

Some other names that Type 2 diabetes goes by:

- Adult-onset diabetes
- Noninsulin-dependence
- Childhood obesity is related as well.
- Impaired Fasting Glucose (prediabetes)
- Impaired Glucose Tolerance (prediabetes)

"Symptoms of Type 2 diabetes often develop slowly—over the course of several years—and can be so mild that you might not even notice them. Many people with Type 2 diabetes have no symptoms" **(REF 29)**.

Because it has already been described well, I would also like to show some quotations from the NIH (National Institute of Diabetes and Digestive and Kidney Diseases) website, Risk Factors for Type 2 diabetes.

These quotes restate what I said earlier, as well as other information on physical activity.

Overweight, obesity, and physical inactivity

"You are more likely to develop Type 2 diabetes if you are not physically active and are overweight or obese. Extra weight sometimes causes insulin resistance and is common in people with Type 2 diabetes. The location of body fat also makes a difference. Extra belly fat is linked to insulin resistance, Type 2 diabetes, and heart and blood vessel disease."

Insulin resistance

"Type 2 diabetes usually begins with insulin resistance, a condition in which muscle, liver, and fat cells do not use insulin well. As a result, your body needs more insulin to help glucose enter cells. At first, the pancreas makes more insulin to keep up with the added demand. Over time, the pancreas can't make enough insulin, and blood glucose levels rise."

Risk Factors for and Prediabetes and Type 2 Diabetes

It is always a great time to get checked for high blood sugar or prediabetes.

Below is a set of Risk Factors for developing Type 2 diabetes, as adapted from the Mayo Clinic literature **(REF 29)**. The literature is also replicated over a number of studies, and publications. It is often difficult to say exactly which factors contribute to the development of Type 2 diabetes. This is why the N-of-1 concept is so important. You may need to develop a specific plan to meet your needs.

However, we do know "risk factors" that correlate to the development of prediabetes and Type 2 diabetes. We also know that if we can control obesity, we are more likely to be able to control prediabetes and Type 2 diabetes. Thus, if we understand the risk factors, specifically the ones we can control, we can make choices to help us avoid these conditions.

Risk Factors for Prediabetes and Type 2 Diabetes

Below is a list of risk factors from both the NIH (National Institute of Diabetes and Digestive and Kidney Diseases) and the NIH (National Heart, Lung, and Blood Institute). **(REF 29, 30)**.

- Overweight or obese
- Age forty-five or older
- Family history of diabetes
- African American, Alaska Native, American Indian, Asian American, Hispanic/Latino, Native Hawaiian, or Pacific Islander
- High blood pressure
- Lack of sleep
- Low level of HDL ("good") cholesterol, or a high level of triglycerides
- History of gestational diabetes or gave birth to a baby weighing nine pounds or more
- Not physically active
- History of heart disease or stroke
- Depression
- Polycystic Ovary Syndrome, also called PCOS
- Have acanthosis (dark, thick, and velvety skin around your neck or armpits)

A specific risk factor is obesity; we reviewed the Body Mass Index (BMI) as a tool to describe the level of obesity. If you have a BMI of twenty-five or higher you are at a higher risk for developing prediabetes or Type 2 diabetes. Remember, the choice is yours for deciding what you do with this information.

Health Problems Associated with Type 2 Diabetes

Obesity is a major risk factor for all sorts of diseases including Type 2 diabetes. If you consume less high-carbohydrate content food, you will be less likely to become obese. And if you are not obese, then you will have a much lower risk of developing diseases, including diabetes.

The complications to your health associated with Type 2 diabetes include:

- Cardiovascular issues
- High blood pressure

- High cholesterol
- Heart disease
- Stroke
- Kidney disease
- Blindness
- Amputations

If the disease continues to progress, several other body functions will shut down.

Stress and Diabetes

Stress linked to eating foods with added sugar for comfort is another part of the disease that is often overlooked.

When you are stressed, do you reach for a soda, candy, chocolate, or a high-sugar-content, flavorful, caffeine-laced sugar-bomb? In my experience, I have seen many people hide their stress by taking comfort in sugar. You can literally see the pleasure release on a person's face as they consume the sugar. The reason we feel that reward sensation is because humans living prior to 350 years ago rarely had access to sugar. The body needs sugar for energy, and before loads of sugar were introduce into common society, the human body developed a feedback loop to give us a quick dopamine release to say, "Good job. You found some sugar. If you find more, you live, and you will get the pleasure sensation again." It's a genuine chemical feedback loop in our bodies, and it's something that many people are not aware of. We discussed these effects in the last chapter.

The good news is that we can avoid or reverse a prediabetes diagnosis.

Preventing Diabetes

Our bodies are amazing! But we really need to think about the excess foods that we put in our bodies. The following excerpt was adapted from the Mayo Clinic's Website **(REF 28)**:

"Healthy lifestyles can help you prevent Type 2 diabetes. Even if you have diabetes in your family, diet and exercise can help you prevent the disease. If you've already received a diagnosis of diabetes, you can use healthy lifestyle choices to help prevent complications. And if you have prediabetes, lifestyle changes can slow or halt the progression from prediabetes to diabetes."

There is no cure for Type 2 diabetes when the disease fully takes hold. If you are diagnosed with Type 2 diabetes, you will be assigned a diet and prescribed physical activity. In the spirit and purpose of this book, I hope that you find some fun activities to do so you won't have to be *prescribed* specific activities. If conditions persist, you will need to take medication. Many people do not like taking medication based on its side effects. In the stories section (Chapter 3), people were looking to avoid having to take pills to manage a disease. When given the option of pills versus nutrition/physical activity, most everyone will take the second choice.

My hope is that this book's message will lessen the likelihood of a Type 2 diabetes diagnosis. I have many "Boomer Generation" friends who live with Type 2 diabetes and manage their symptoms through the use of medication, nutrition, and exercise. But there are side effects to taking any drug. If we can, we really would like to escape the disease by looking to change our diets before a prediabetes diagnosis. I would like to see the statistics regarding the prevalence of prediabetes and Type 2 diabetes cases by age group; will there be more Gen Xers with prediabetes per capita in comparison to the Baby Boomer Generation?

Eat Healthy Foods, Get Physical, Lose Excess Pounds

Exercise will burn excess sugar in the bloodstream to help lower the amount of sugar in your blood. Healthcare providers should provide you with a regimen of exercises to help mitigate the effects of the disease. Part 3 of this book is dedicated to what physical activity should be performed on a daily basis.

The American Diabetes Association recommends at least 150 minutes of moderate activity per week: walking, bike riding, or swimming five times a week for thirty-minute sessions, at a minimum **(REF 31)**. This is also mirrored by the NIH **(REF 32)**.

Working out will:

- Lower blood glucose levels
- Lower blood pressure
- Improve blood flow
- Burn extra calories to help keep weight down
- Improve mood
- Possibly help you sleep better

What we need to focus on is how we are going to execute our N-of-1 Challenge to prevent a diagnosis that we don't want. The next part of this book will present information and lists of different activities that can be performed

Professionals to Contact and Other Resources

The amount of literature and information about prediabetes and Type 2 diabetes can be overwhelming. As part of this project, I have created a website (www.nof1challenge.com) devoted to sharing the most up-to-date information. On my website, you'll find a blog with links to some of the best literature and organizations to contact. There are several great organizations that prepare summaries of data from clinical research and real-world action items. Some of these organizations have already been referenced during this section.

- The Mayo Clinic
- Harvard Medical School
- The Diabetes Association
- The National Institute of Diabetes and Digestive and Kidney Disease
- The National Institute of Health
- Centers for Disease Control and Prevention
- Medical schools and local universities

However, as a reminder, this book is not designed to replace the experience of speaking with a medical doctor, Registered Dietitian (RD), or a Certified Diabetes Educator (CDE). This book is designed to help with awareness, to help educate, and to provide sources for you to seek extra guidance. Many types of coaches or specialists are helpful, but you have to be ready to listen to your coach and provide feedback so the coach can adjust personalized plans as necessary.

The N-of-1 Challenge and a Quick Review for Nutrition

We have covered several different topics with regards to nutrition, carbohydrate consumption, and obesity-related diseases in Part 2 of this book. First, we looked at the chemistry of different molecules and defined what we mean by simple and complex carbohydrates. Then we discussed the glycemic index as a tool for understanding the properties of different foods and how they interact with our bodies. From there, we moved into a discussion on body mass index, calorie counting, and the history of sugar consumption. Finally, we looked at different diseases that are associated with obesity. Specifically, we covered prediabetes and Type 2 diabetes. We have covered several pieces of information, now what should we do?

For my particular N-of-1 Challenge, I have adopted a more "practical paleo" type diet than is currently common in society. I have also excluded wheat-based foods (bread, pasta, beer, etc.), dairy, and food that had added sugar. Also, I do have days where I enjoy cheesecake, other sweets, or fried chicken. I will enjoy a beer every once in a while—I love getting together with friends and having a beer—but I can only have one or two of particular types of beers. If I go past that, or if I drink one of those "no-go" beers, I get sick and feel terrible. Over the last five years, I have really tailored my diet to my personal N-of-1.

Another factor for your N-of-1 Challenge and plan should be to include an investigation on food sensitivities, intolerances, and allergies. For example, I have several acquaintances who have eliminated certain types of peppers from their diets because of acid reflux symptoms. As I mentioned earlier, I had to cut wheat products out of my diet. Although not fully recognized, wheat sensitivity and intolerance have become somewhat common in society. For me, my wheat sensitivity has created a situation where giving up bread, pasta, and beer has been much easier than I thought it would be. Although not a major theme in this book,

I strongly suggest that you look at food sensitivities, intolerances, and allergies that you may have. Acknowledging a food sensitivity may also be important to help with your overall health.

When we learn what our own N-of-1 diet should be, we feel better and we are probably going to be healthier. For example, I don't have cheese or milk, because that just makes me feel better. I still, on occasion, have milk in coffee, but I have eliminated it most of the time. I still have cheese at times, but it is not an everyday occurrence. For some people, they don't need to give up cheese or milk, but they may not need to give up other types of foods. For each of us, there are several factors that can contribute to an improved diet.

What is your N-of-1 diet?

How to Change Your Diet

During my N-of-1 Challenge, I tried a ketogenic diet. For this type of diet, I highly recommend supervision. You can make yourself sick if you are not monitoring this diet properly. The list of foods that I ate while losing weight was not 100% ketogenic, but I did rapidly drop weight to a point where I became unhealthy. I became too skinny and my immune system did not function properly. After performing this diet, I readjusted to a diet that can be called carb-restricted, not carb-eliminated. Now, I get most of the "carbs" that I need from rice, sweet potatoes, and other "clean" sources. I perform eight to ten hours per week of "hard physical activities," so my diet needs are much different than when I started my N-of-1 Challenge. There are modified diets depending on how athletic you are -if you reach that level - if you want to.

However, the point of this chapter is: *we must cut the excess sugar and carbohydrates out of our diets so that we do not become obese.* The simple calorie-counting exercise reviewed in the previous section should illustrate the math related to food intake. This is a great tool to help you change your diet. We only need to consume a certain amount of food for the energy we burn each day, and we need to eat low glycemic index foods that also have more nutritional value. Your N-of-1 diet should start with the elimination of certain low-value carbohydrates and certain added-sugar items. The glycemic index is also a great tool for helping with dietary choices.

Another difficult but incredibly beneficial step is to reduce portion sizes at dinner. This is often easier said than done. All you need to do is simply reduce food portions, and your stomach will catch up with you. At first, it may be painful but stick with it.

Plan to eat half the carbs you typically have during a week—half as much bread, half as many servings of potatoes, etc. Keep your protein intake the same. I also suggest reducing the amount of red meat by one-third and replacing it with another source of protein (fish, chicken, eggs, pork, lamb, etc.)

Electronic Journaling of Food – The Best Practice

As I progressed through my N-of-1 Challenge, I found that electronic journaling was the best tool for helping me lose weight. I could track and see how many carbs I was eating. Many electronic journals and apps have templates and "pre-entries" to choose from, e.g. hamburgers at certain restaurants, eggs and bacon for breakfast, pasta and beer at dinner, or that bag of chips or delicious ice cream you snack on at night. But once again, with any journal, these are just tools. If you miss an entry, you might as well not use the app.

The only way to regain a healthy lifestyle is through achievable goals and accountability. Some of my current favorite electronic journals include: My Fitness Pal, Lose It! SparkPeople, and Fooducate. There are actually several new electronic journals available since the conception of this book.

At first, just observe what you eat all week. Record what you are eating in a journal and observe the number of calories that you are consuming. Make sure to include all the sauces and snacks, too. After seeing where you are, adjust your diet so that you eliminate some of the extra carb sources. This is a step that must happen if you want to get your diet under control. You have to pay attention to what you are eating before you can know what you need to change. This is how you can set goals and map the results by collecting data on the food that you eat.

For my story, it took another four to eight months to fully get this under control. Some of the foods I thought were good for me were *not*. Dried fruit, I quickly learned, actually has hundreds of grams of sugar— not much different than a candy bar and more calories than a bag of chips! I also learned that it is easy to find a justification to "cheat" if you are not careful. That is why journaling is so important. Use a detailed journal, or you will not get the benefits of its use.

The next step is to understand the importance of core strength and physical activity. When we are active, we burn glucose in the blood. Thus, physical activity can help us regulate our blood sugar **(REF 32)**. Part 3 of this book contains ample information on core-strength and physical activities.

Before moving into Part 3 of this book, I want to cover an interesting topic. Have you heard about the microbiome and its emerging research?

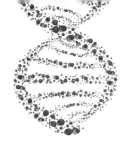

CHAPTER 7:

NEW CUTTING-EDGE RESEARCH AND THE MICROBIOME

Before jumping into the next part on core strength, I want to discuss something called the microbiome—something I see as cutting edge, modern, and fun. This is a topic of health that may change the way that we approach certain diseases. The microbiome is important with the way in which it interacts with our bodies as related to human health. In fact, I feel that it is one of the most fascinating trends and topics in biotechnology today—specifically, for its importance in the environment and for human health.

We are living during a phase of history when an extraordinary amount of new information is being accumulated about the microbes that live inside and on all of us—good and bad microbiota. These microbes are essential to our survival and can even make us sick if we have the wrong populations in our stomach and intestines.

The microbiome is comprised of the millions of different types of bacteria that live among us. There are trillions of different microbes in the world, some helpful and others harmful. They live in our water, inside our bodies, on and in our pets, in our carpet, on our computer, in our kitchen, and just about everywhere else.

For a more specific definition, the microbes—or the microbiota—that live in these specific environments include viruses, fungi, protists, archaea, and bacteria. For the purposes of this book, I want to create two types of awareness. First, that the microbiome exists and second, that there are bacteria that we need to live that help us with nutrition and food digestion.

Helpful vs. Harmful Bacteria

We know that we can contract various infections that will make us sick and cause us great problems. But we often don't think of bacteria as being helpful. As is the case with many other "yin and yang" trade-offs in life, there are bacteria that are important to us for maintaining life and helping us maintain a healthy lifestyle. Some of the latest research in this area has directly linked diseases to good and bad populations of gut microbes in our digestive tracts. Much of this research is cutting edge, and new information continues to be generated on the topic. I will share just a few of the more interesting, phenomenal research results that have been reported in regard to nutrition and human disease.

One quick note, of all the drugs on the market produced for humans, over half of all pharmaceuticals come from microbiota. I started my career working on projects related to "Natural Products," or the molecules created by plants, animals, or microbiota that could be isolated and used for their pharmaceutical properties. The philosophy is that nature "has been doing this a long time" and much of what we need for our own health can be found in nature. Apply this logic to nutrition.

From a biochemical standpoint, we have only explored about 1% of chemistry from the full population of the microbiota. Unfortunately, it is hard to keep many of them alive in the lab after extracting them from their natural habitats. We have made great progress over the last five years; however, as a community, we are spending more time and money on gut microbiome research.

New research reveals links between nutrition and healthy vs. non-healthy bacteria. For example, we know (or have known) that there are certain gut bacteria that are important for producing Vitamins K and B. We also know that gut microbes are important for immune function. Infant microbiota are influenced by breastfeeding, and we have found that a broader diversity of good microbe types leads to improved health.

Gut microbes live in the mucus found in the intestines and work together with the rest of our bodies to keep us healthy **(REF 33)**. Current research is also revealing that certain types of microbes in our bodies contribute to pain, mood, sleep, stress, and immune response as related to nutrition. Also, the microbiome has been found to vary among individuals due to factors such as climate, hygiene, age, gender, genetic disposition, and diet **(REF 34)**.

To quickly summarize, the body and mind can be affected by the microbiome found living in your intestines, stomach, and other parts of your body. Generally, these are the ways in which the microbiome affects us:

• Nutrition
• Sleep and mood
• Inflammation and infection
• Skin
• Regulating the immune system
• Balancing blood sugar
• Absorption of nutrients
• Calming emotions

Based on the research from the last decade, "gut microbe health" has been implicated in several disease areas, including:

• Obesity
• Cancer
• Mental health
• Autism
• Alzheimer's
• Diabetes

The purpose of this Chapter is to quickly show where current research is with regard to health and the microbiome. With a change in diet and reaching a N-of-1 Goal, we will also improve our own microbiome in our guts. It follows that the same consideration taken for diet, reduced sugar, and/or exercise will help maintain healthy microbe populations in our symbiotic relationship. For example, you may not be getting enough fiber for your "healthy gut microbes". Fiber helps with a diverse, "healthy microbiome", and this diversity generally means improved gut health.

A publication from the NIH states, "Healthy adult humans each typically harbor more than 1,000 species of bacteria belonging to a relatively few known bacterial phyla with Bacteroidetes and Firmicutes being the dominant phyla. The microbiota of the gut is quite diverse compared to other body sites, and there is considerable variation in the constituents of the gut microbiota among apparently healthy individuals. As a way of accounting for the microbial variability among healthy individuals, researchers have tried to identify certain stable patterns of microbial populations in the human population" **(REF 34).**

The NIH manuscript continues on to discuss the different types of microbes that have been identified and categorized, and there are some great profiles of healthy and bad gut microbes. If you would like to follow up on more gut microbe information, I have posted the information for your review on the www.nof1challenge.com website. Below, I have pulled some of the key information from the report.

Key Points from the NIH Microbiome Manuscript

"An individual's microbiome is quite stable over time, but there is variability at the extremes of age and among different individuals. Diet and other environmental factors also affect the composition of the microbiome" **(REF 34)**.

"In comparison to healthy controls, alterations in the microbiota are recognized in a growing number of disease states, but outside of Clostridium difficile infection, the role of these microbiota alterations in the pathogenesis of disease is uncertain. A better understanding of the functional interactions between the human host and the microbiome is very likely to lead to new diagnostic, prognostic and therapeutic capabilities" **(REF 34)**.

In regard to our N-of-1 concept, research has found that almost two-thirds of microbes can be unique to individuals. In the research that I have seen and studied, it seems as though there is a link between poor health and an increased number of microbes that primarily use sugar and carbohydrates.

In the end, it's what you put in your body that is important to having a healthy microbe population in your intestinal tract. If you eat the proper food, you will most likely receive the nutrients that you need for a healthy gut microbiome. This leads back to tools like the glycemic index and glycemic load. Apply this philosophy and it may automatically improve your gut health. Supplements are also available to help increase the population of healthy colonies living in your body.

This was a relatively short chapter; however, my goal is to create awareness of the microbiome before moving onto the next topic of "Core Strength, Mobility, and Physical Activity." Remember, the food you eat is also used by the microbiome in your gut for their growth and contribute to your overall health.

PART 3:

CORE STRENGTH, MOBILITY, AND PHYSICAL ACTIVITY: YOUR N-OF-1 CHALLENGE

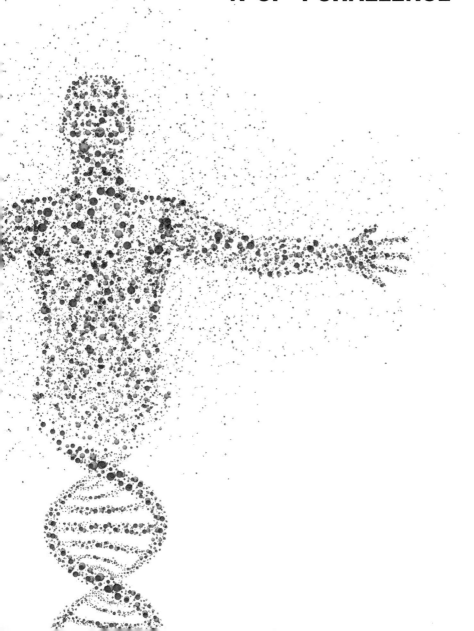

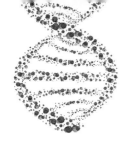

CHAPTER 8:

CORE STRENGTH AND MOBILITY

In this part of the book, we are going to expand on several import-ant topics related to physical activity and maintaining a healthy life-style. We all know that we need to stay physically active to maintain our health. As we've discussed, physical activity is one of the best ways to lessen risk factors for many diseases, including prediabetes and Type 2 diabetes. This part of the book focuses on different aspects of core strength and exercises that will help you lose weight and reduce your risk factors. As we mentioned at the beginning of this book, we have to pay attention to both our nutrition and core strength.

For me, I was able to change my diet easily and was able to re-strengthen my core muscles over time. Six years ago, I was in chronic back, shoulder, and neck pain. I was barely functional. As well, I was 55 pounds heavier than I am now. I went to a shoulder specialist, but he said that there was nothing wrong with my shoulder. I thought that I had a rotator cuff injury from years of baseball and sports abuse. After this positive diagnosis, I was not sure what the problem was. I decided to visit Dr. Dex Alvarez based on a local recommendation that he may be able to help. He is a chiropractor that practices more of a holistic view of health. He looks at all aspects of lifestyle and health, not just focusing on one area or medicine.

Dex performed his assessment, started working on my back and recommended some stretches. I did not know it, but I had a nagging hip injury that was actually the source of the pain and irritation. People said that I had walked with a limp for many years, but I did not really take notice of it. Because of the pain in my shoulder, I thought this was the problem, but it was actually my hip, along with some spinal issues that had started to take hold. After a month of changing my behavior and starting to stretch more, my hip joint slipped in and out of joint, causing my hip flexor muscle group to go into spasm. This resulted in some of the worst pain I have had in my life—much worse than all the broken noses from my reckless abandoned style of play. I could not move for three days.

This took six months to get over; however, when it was all over, my chronic pain had subsided. I stuck with my stretching regimen, and my body healed. I had to pay very close attention to my workout regimen during the early period. I had a combination of several issues. My hip had been partially locked in for years. My spine was starting to twist, I had three vertebrates that were on their way to compression, I had muscle shortening because of the amount of sitting and traveling, and finally, I was overweight. My knees hurt as well. Fun fact: Every pound of excess weight exerts about four pounds of extra pressure on the knees.

I had visited many doctors before, but Dr. Alvarez provided the proper assessment and treatment needed. Dex is a chiropractor that looks at the whole patient while providing treatment, as well as offer other advice. Not only does Dex look at the central nervous system (CNS), but he works on nutrition and habit-forming behaviors. In my opinion, Dex represents a growing class of practitioners—those who look at patients holistically, thus finding and fixing the underlying problem for that particular individual. This does not mean that he fixes *everything*. He will refer patients to other specialists as needed. However, in the end, he looks at the person as a whole. During the last part of this book, I interview Dr. Dex and discuss his philosophies on preventive medicine.

Mobility is very important and essential to health. It is an over-looked lifestyle aspect. To help shed more light on this concept, I interviewed

Dr. Alyssa Stewart, an expert in mobility and balancing muscle group strength. She can essentially customize workouts to help people regain proper mobility. At times, there are common muscle groups that will need to be stretched in order to alleviate something called muscle shorting. Muscle shorting—or possible overuse injuries—can pull on joints, causing pain and discomfort.

Among many mobility topics, Dr. Stewart is an expert in providing therapy for individuals who have not been active for long periods of time. What I find most interesting about her philosophies is that we can often alleviate pain with proper stretching, training, and exercise. She also has advice for those that are overactive and injure themselves from pushing too hard. During the interview, I worked to stay on task within the themes of this book—nutrition, core strength, and mind-space. The goal is to help provide options to improve your own mobility to add to your N-of-1 Challenge.

The Importance of Mobility and Core Strength— An Interview with Dr. Alyssa Stewart

When performing interviews, it is good to prepare. This interview was interesting because I was under the impression that Dr. Stewart mostly treated patients involved in car crashes and other accidents. As it turned out, my thoughts on her practice were not completely correct. It is good to keep an open mind to new information and to let go of some pre-conceived notions.

This is where I started the conversation with Alyssa: I have read and researched that you are a mobility expert. Can you please let us know what sorts of injuries you treat and the importance of mobility and core strength?

Normally, nine out of ten of the injuries that I treat are due to over- or under-use of a muscle group. I don't really treat that many traumatic accidents. The most common injuries that I treat include (1) low back pain (2) shoulders and knees, and (3) ankles and hands. They are so dysfunctional; the joints are actually pulled on by the dysfunctional muscle.

An overuse injury could be a baseball pitcher who has thrown a couple million pitches or someone that has been sitting in a chair for ten hours at a time for several years.

Overuse injuries are often not from a tear or ligament damage. For example, many people have come to me with low back pain. They didn't tear anything. It's just that the muscles have become so dysfunctional and tight that they're pulling on the joints in ways they should not be pulled on. That is the source of the pain. Patients are having pain at the point where the muscle inserts into that joint after years of chronic tightness and dysfunction. One side of the muscle group is weak, and the muscle group on the other side is super tight. Over time, this leads to pain.

Conservatively, mobility training can help provide relief for pain. It's a combination of mobility exercises, stretching, stability exercises, strengthening, and motor control exercises. It's just learning how to manage the body again. For example, if you sit all day, it will cause your hip flexors and thoracic spine to get locked down and tight. You have to reverse this shortening by performing exercises and stretching daily. It's not going to be fixed overnight. This is not a quick fix. The quick fix is taking a pill or surgery—if that gives you any type of fix—but that could just lead to more issues. Putting Band-Aids on problems will never solve them. But we all have something that we tend to default to, and it's about learning what that is and working on it.

When healing from an injury that needs extensive physical training, how do you help the patient maintain a positive outlook for the recovery? How do you keep a patient on track when you're working through several months of exercise?

It's the same way when we speak about fad diets. If you tell someone they'll lose thirty pounds in two weeks, that's obviously not going to last. After that, they will go right back to whatever they were doing because there is no change in habit. When I work with clients, I train them into understanding that it's not for a certain time—it has to be a lifestyle change. I teach them that they need to pay attention to how their muscle feels when they perform a certain exercise or stretch. I don't just tell them to do these three exercises. I teach the client to also pay attention to the response from the exercise.

The more I can educate the patient on what they need to do and why they need to do it, the more likely they are to do it. If someone understands that because they sit all day, their hip flexors are going to get tight, along with their back, then I can teach them exactly what they need for helping those muscle groups.

If I'm able to teach someone, they are less likely to re-enter the initial program. The more they want to know about muscle groups, joints, and mobility, the more likely they're going to be successful with their program.

Patients have the same injury again, and they come right back in the system. This is because they are discharged once they are pain-free (have regained basic function). This does not mean they are actually fully functional. The money for preventative care can often not be there. So, once they re-injure themselves, they can get an insurance payment again. It is difficult for insurance to cover these people. Preventative care is just not present.

People ask, "How long do I need to do this for?" I reply, "How much longer are you going to brush your teeth?" Every day. Typically, for the rest of your life. So, if you want your body to work and to be pain-free, you should do something to work on it for the rest of your life.

Also, most people don't come to me unless they are in pain. No one ever visits me and says that they're worried that they might be in pain someday because their hip flexors are bad. They wait until the pain strikes. They come in here, hobbling, wanting me to fix them because they have a CrossFit tournament tomorrow.

Could you elaborate more on what you do and where your philosophies come from?

I do the same assessment for everyone. It's a functional movement screen, and I look at how your body is functioning from the top of your head to your foot. Based on that information, I start deciding what we need to work on.

None of this was invented by me. One of the sources I use is called the "Joint by Joint" approach. It's a book that discusses how, with every major joint in our body, we go from mobility to stability. If you look at the ankle, the ankle tends to be too tight, and thus, we need to stretch it. The hip tends to be too tight, and thus, we need to mobilize it. Our joints go through these alternating lack-mobility then lack-stability, all the way up our bodies. If we look at the ones that are lacking mobility, it's our ankles, our hips, and our thoracic spine. It's our shoulder joints, and then it's our wrists. These are the joints that can often lack mobility and will cause dysfunction. On the flip side, all those joints between our knees, lumbar spine, mid-neck, and scapula region—if we don't stabilize those, we're going to cause dysfunction.

If I were to look at the three most important stretches for people who sit at a desk, it would be your hip flexors, your thoracic spine, and your shoulder joint. It could also be your wrists, depending on if you use a mouse all day.

Besides just sitting at a desk, I think the majority of us tend to be too tight. We need to work on mobility and stretching. But there are a few of us—I'm one of those people—who happen to be hypermobile. Thus, I have to work on stability exercises. But most people are generally too tight. It's important to make sure that you are performing the correct exercises.

This goes into the whole education part—learning what your body needs, understanding it, and then working on it.

I'm curious about how you manage the stress from the job. How do you manage absorbing patients' energy? How do you maintain your own mind-space?

Everyone can handle certain limits. Health care providers are often empathetic, and this is what makes us good at our jobs. We really do feel and care. And because we feel and care, there is a limit to what we can handle. In the end, we have to recognize what our own personal limit is for a certain discipline and listen to advice. During the week, I work out and enjoy playing with my pets. I also speak to a therapist once a month. That helps, and I also work to reset the mind. If you feel empty inside, or bitter, how can you be helpful to your patients?

Dr. Stewart's views on mobility are valuable. Are there any points from this conversation that you find relevant to you and your N-of-1 goals? Is mobility where you should start your N-of-1 Challenge? I had to start here—stretching and balancing my muscle groups. I had to strengthen my back muscles before I could move into my next goal of strength training.

"Sitting is the New Smoking" – Activities that Can Lead to Overuse Pain

Sitting might seem like an unlikely source of injury, but in reality, it is one of the leading causes of pain. Let's start with what sitting does to our muscles and joints over time. For one thing, a seated position cuts off circulation; it is not a natural position for humans to maintain.

We can make fun of the ergonomic training our company requires, but there is useful information from this kind of education. Personally, I can no longer use a mouse with a computer or sit at a lab bench for too long. I get sharp pains in my upper right back and shoulder. Sometimes, I have to get therapeutic massages to keep my shoulder loose. In the gym, I can lift weights without feeling any pain in that area or adding any new problems. However, sitting at a desk for hours at a time can put me back into deep pain again if I'm not paying attention to my posture and taking breaks. For my own N-of-1 plan, I now use a stand-up desk at times and rotate between sitting and standing while I work. This has been incredibly helpful for keeping my muscles stretched out and in much less pain.

If you sit for a long period of time, here are some quick suggestions from the NIH (National Institute of Diabetes and Kidney Disease). This is a simple list of exercises to do so that you may help mitigate future problems and pain:

Perform 3 minutes of exercise for every 30 minutes of sitting **(REF 32)**. This could include leg lifts or extensions, overhead arm stretches, desk chair swivels, torso twists, side lunges, or walking in place. In general, if you sit for too long, try to perform a 30-minute break of aerobic exercise each day, most days of the week.

For the rest of this chapter, I will cover different types of stretches and exercises that can be used to help with mobility and counteract unhealthy activities such as sitting for long periods of time. Please remember that this book does not intend to be used as a substitute for professional care for previous injuries. The suggestions here do not account for acute injuries (accidents, broken bones, torn muscles, ligament damage, etc.). Before adding core workouts or a new stretching regimen, please consult a specialist or doctor.

We don't want to make our N-of-1 Challenge goals too difficult to reach. If you need to, get a coach to help you set goals.

Stretching and Foam Rolling

Stretching and foam rolling are two of the most common activities used to prevent muscle shortening. In this section, we are only covering the mobility aspect of health. We will cover cardio health during the next chapter and core and strength training two chapters from now.

Stretching

This is where I started my recovery. Learning to perform my stretches every day turned out to be very important as I worked to improve my health. Stretching really helped me regain the flexibility that I had lost from sitting at desks and performing repetitive tasks at the bench in the lab. If you sit for long periods of time—at a desk, on a plane, or in an automobile—you may have muscle shortening issues, certain compressed joints, and vertebrae. Stretching does not have to take long. I find time for 15 to 30 minutes per day.

There are many resources on the internet that describe and illustrate different stretches that you can perform. In Appendix 2, I have some photographs of example stretches for you to check out. We will have suggested stretches for you to view, as well as videos on the www. nof1challenge.com website. We can all benefit from improved mobility with a stretching routine.

Foam Rolling

At times, we need to soften muscles and improve circulation. Foam rolling helps to keep your muscles softer to prevent them from tightening up.

Foam rolling involves a foam tube (**Figure 3**) that is used by "rolling" a set muscle group. **Appendix 2** illustrates a few of the exercises that can be performed while foam rolling. To perform the exercise, you simply roll back and forth on a certain choice muscle group. We will also have review information for the exercises on the www.nof1challenge.com website.

Often, injuries occur when muscles are too tight. This is different than the lactic acid "burn" that we feel after a hard-cardio workout. Foam rolling helps break up adhesions and scar tissue and speed up the healing and recovery process after your workout. This can help prevent muscle cramps and can to help to avoid injury.

Side note: As part of your nutrition N-of-1 Challenge, you should also be drinking more water. We mentioned this during the nutrition section. Since we are going to eliminate sugar water, we need to replace it with something. I typically only drink water and coffee during the week. Hydration is vital to the prevention of muscle cramps and injuries. It also helps with healing and clearing toxins while you work out.

Of all the stretches and maintenance I perform, foam rolling is probably my least favorite. But I have found it to be a key element of muscle maintenance. The goal of foam rolling is to prevent muscle shortening.

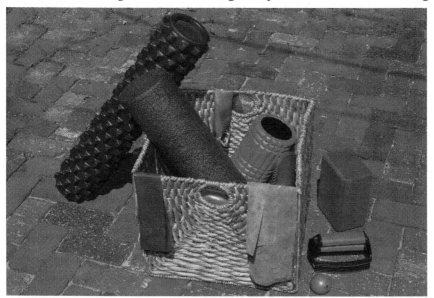

Figure 3 - Examples of Foam Rollers along with another workout equipment.

Mobility and stretching are important to overall health. Daily stretching can be a great place to start before attempting a workout program. Mobility is where I started before reaching the consistent workout plan that I have now. Are you going to add these elements to your N-of-1 Challenge?

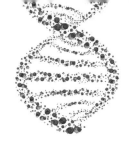

CHAPTER 9:
CARDIO AND ZONE TRAINING

Many people dislike the thought of cardio workouts. However, there are numerous types of exercises and workout plans available for all types of individuals. There is an endless combination of workout plans that can be tweaked to arrive at what works best for your N-of-1 Challenge.

Changing your diet alone will not result in a complete transformation. We linked this thought to nutrition in Chapter 6 and how to mitigate risk factors associated with obesity. As we discussed in Chapter 8, humans were not designed to sit at desks all day or constantly lack physical activity. We developed as hunters and gatherers to obtain nutrition. We did not drive to our local food mart to pick out what we would eat. We had to hunt and collect what we ate. Since we do live in a today's society, we need to spend the extra time getting the exercise that we need.

I will classify four major exercises in this book for discussion. This does not include the topic of stretching or yoga type exercises. Stretching was included in the mobility section before this chapter. Make sure that stretching is part of your regimen and allow 20 to 30 minutes for this type of activity. As mentioned before, stretching is often where we start before attempting a workout program, depending on where you are in health. Yoga is definitely a physical activity; however, yoga brings other benefits to help manage mind-space. Thus, yoga is covered in Part 4 of this book.

Our four classifications of workouts for goal setting include:

1. Heart Rate Zone Training
2. Strength Gain Training
3. Core Strength Training and Powerlifting
4. Outdoor and Recreational Training

Your current level of health will dictate what sort of exercise you should choose from, and your N-of-1 Challenge will change as you reach new goals. After four years of working on my core strength, I have rotated through all four types of training. I still rotate through them, and I find that a variety of exercises are fun and stimulating.

Just to reiterate, if you have suffered any kind of injury in the past, it is best to consult with a professionally licensed trainer. Not all trainers are the same. Different trainers have different specialties. It is best to shop and ask around before deciding on the best trainer to help you get the ball rolling.

Zone Training and Cardio

Where I started with my recovery is not where I ended up in my current N-of-1 Challenge. I have completed the recovery goals of my challenge, and now maintain a schedule to preserve the balance that I have reached. I started my recovery by simply walking for one or two miles. As my core strength improved over time, I moved into more rigorous cardio training. Eventually, I found something called Heart Rate Zone training.

This type of training can be applied to any sort of cardio training—jogging, swimming, or cycling. It can also be applied to any sort of indoor training machines that involve cardio. It is not just limited to cycling, my personal example in this chapter.

I personally love Heart Rate Zone training; it has allowed me to deepen my connection with my body and muscle groups while I train. If you have not heard of this type of scheme, our heart rate, for training purposes, can be split into five zones. The idea is that different benefits are realized during training at different heart rates within those five zones. Each one of these zones will be based on the percent maximum heart rate (MHR). At each heart rate zone, your body burns different percentages of fat, protein, and carbohydrates (**Table 4**). The goal is to maintain a certain heart rate in a zone to reach a goal. For example, if you want to burn fat, work within Zone 1 or 2. I found Heart Rate Zone training to be very valuable in improving overall health. For example, I was out of energy after a twenty-minute bike ride when I started my training. Now I can ride up to five or six hours when I perform cycling events.

If you would like to perform this sort of training, I suggest that you purchase a heart rate monitor. I think that many of the modern watches that people purchase now collect this sort of data. If your watch does not collect this data, you can purchase a device to do so. This will allow you to monitor the "type" of calories that you are burning—all dependent on what your heart rate is. Once you start this type of training, pay attention to how you feel and the results. This is how I made new connections with my body—working to maintain a certain heart rate for different intervals for different results.

Zone	MHR	Intensity	Training Type	Burn
1	50 to 60%	Low	Walking, a light hike	Carbs: 10% Protein: 5% Fat: 85%
2	60 to 70%	Moderate	Faster-paced walking or hiking burns increased calories per minute	Carbs: 10% Protein: 5% Fat: 85%
3	70 to 80%	Aerobic Zone	Endurance Training Healthier circulatory system by increasing lung and heart and capacity through new blood vessel growth 20 to 60 minutes for best fitness results	Carbs: 50% Protein: 5% Fat: 50%
4	70 to 80%	Anaerobic Zone	Threshold zone "VO2" maximum (maximal oxygen intake) Improves the amount of oxygen that can be can consumed by the body Lactic acid production Commonly done for 10 to 20 min	Carbs: 85% Protein: <1% Fat: 15%
5	90 to 100%	Red-Line Zone	Hard, high-intensity cardio Most people can't stay at for more than 1 or 2 minutes	Carbs: 90% Protein: <1% Fat: 15%

Table 4 - Heart Rate Zone Training definitions and information.

Cardio Exercises and My N-of-1

The most common types of cardio workouts include walking, hiking, jogging, cycling, and swimming. Personally, I do not find jogging enjoyable. This is why I played baseball. In fact, I have never liked running as an exercise. I also don't enjoy swimming or being in the water. Cycling turned out to be the perfect choice after moving on from my initial mobility and core strength issues.

Four years ago (or about nine months into my recovery), I was deciding on my next hobby: surfing, playing guitar or cycling. In the end, I chose the bike because I knew that it would be a healthy choice. My hip-flexor had just started to feel well again, and I decided that jogging and running would not be good for my inflammation. I was also told to avoid high impact training as my back and hip muscles healed. The new Trek I bought turned out to be a blast! I purchased new clip-in pedals, new shoes, and a Garmin device to track my rides and collect data, and I was all in after four months.

I also learned that I could be competitive in my local area with other cyclists through a software app called STRAVA. Thus, I mixed my new hobby of cycling with my new nutritional knowledge I had gained. That was when I really started to lose the extra pounds, matching what I ate, when I ate, and when I planned to ride my bike or workout.

With regards to zone training, I turned my cycling journey into a training routine and a new habit within four months after purchasing my bike. My average speed per ride was 13.5 mph when I started. After one year, I was averaging 16.5 mph. During my peak two years ago, I was averaging 18 mph over 64 miles with 4,000 feet of climbing. Since my peak performance two years ago, I base my schedule on maintaining a certain weight (my BMI weight of 195 pounds) and my current diet.

My personal example for my N-of-1 is cycling; your cardio sport may be different. You may like swimming, jogging, or going to the gym to use one of the machines. What is important is that you choose some sort of activity. Choose an exercise that you like to do. You are in charge of your N-of-1 Challenge. Don't settle on someone else's definition of the "correct" exercise. You know what you enjoy.

The Importance of Journaling

In the nutrition part of this book, I outlined the benefits of electronic journaling for calorie counting. This practice is also useful for tracking different workout routines and activities.

I prefer to transfer my workout data from STRAVA to an Excel sheet so that I can track them and create accountability. I sit down every five to seven days and review my exercise data. STRAVA provides real-time data to help me maintain my monthly goals. I also record how I felt during the session—great ride, tired legs, worn out from traveling, sore back, etc. Monitoring your body's feedback helps you mitigate the effects of over-training. Recovery time after working out is also important. You don't want to over train and create a new over-use injury.

STRAVA can also be used for a variety of different types of cardio workouts. I have several friends and acquaintances that us this app (or other apps) to record their workouts. We follow each other and support each other through the app. The apps can be used to record whatever sort of workout you want to choose.

To show the power and fun of journaling, I have tracked all of my rides during the last four years. This has helped me keep up with my own personal N-of-1 Challenge. **Figure 4** is the number of miles that I have ridden per day (gym or on the road) plotted over time. What is fun, is that we can see different trends emerge from the data collected.

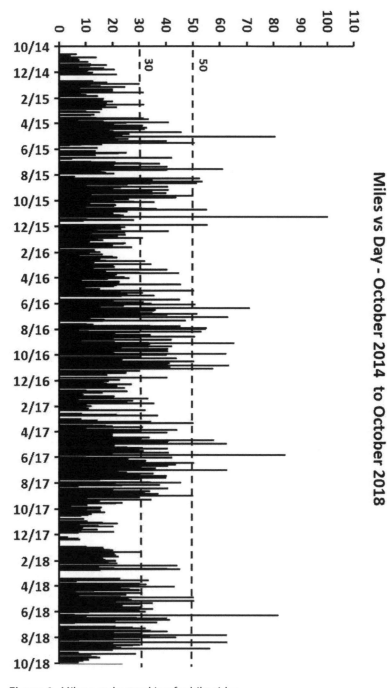

Figure 4 - Miles per day tracking for bike rides.

Most everyone will agree that journaling is one of the most important aspects of tracking our physical activity and nutrition. We may also collect more data than we need. **Figure 4,** for example, simply plots the number of miles that I have ridden per day (gym or road) over time. We see that I have been able to keep up with my weekly, monthly, and yearly goals for cycling and cardio. Looking closer at the data, we can see a gap in the data (over a week) that represents days that I did not ride. This correlates to some sort of event. For this particular piece of data, it is related to being sick, traveling, or some other event that prevented me from staying on schedule. If you get off schedule for one week, don't let it go to two weeks. Get back at it as soon as possible.

Another interesting piece of information from the data is my seasonal "biorhythm" while living in Tennessee for three years. I am not an expert in biorhythm, but I do have years of general interpretation of data analysis. The trend is easy to see; during the winter, there was no way I could cycle outside, as my body does not work under 60 degrees Fahrenheit. My body had a hard time in the gym during the winter as well. I grew up in Florida and moved to Tennessee about four years ago. I moved back home to Florida in March of 2018. As I adapt back to the environment here, I look forward to seeing how my body reacts to the Florida winter. I look forward to seeing how my N-of-1 changes and how I adapt to a new program.

The data in the bar chart only shows how many miles I traveled during a bike ride. This does not show speed, heart rate, or other detailed information. Many people wear devices such as Fitbits or Garmin to monitor their fitness, but how many actually *analyze* all that data? A walking/steps-per-day goal is a great place to start, but you should also make plans to move to the next step in health besides just counting steps. Remember, data is only as useful when you know what to do with it.

Through collecting years of data and journaling your workouts, you can find out more about yourself than you know now. However, until you start collecting data on your workouts, you will not be able to track your goals or make decisions on what to change.

Suggested Cardio Workout Schedules

The below suggested cardio workout plan can be applied to any sort of cardio exercise. We can apply this plan to jogging, cycling, swimming, or exercises on machines in gyms. The time and heart rate zones are taken from NIH guidance's referenced in Chapter 6 **(REF 5)**. When performing Heart Rate Zone Training, it can be hard to hold your rate constant when you first start. But as with all things, you will get better with time.

Currently, a typical week of cardio training for me looks like the following:

Day	Zone	Notes on Exercise
Day 1:	Z2/Z3	1-hour cardio
Day 2:	Rest Day	A rest day can be just as important as a workout day.
Day 3:	Z2/Z3, Z4/Z5	45-minute cardio with intervals: 5-minutes in Z2/Z3 2-minutes Z4/Z5 Repeated for duralon of workout
Day 4:	Rest Day	
Day 5:	Choose Zone Profile	2-hour bike ride, choosing a zone profile
Day 6:	Z2/Z3	45-minute - 2-hour
Day 7:	Rest Day	
Note: Day Six and Day Seven are interchangeable, and the ride times may vary depending on the circumstance		

Table 5 - Base cardio workout schedule for stating and intermediate programs

The start of your N-of-1 Cardio work-out plan will be dictated on you current activity level. I suggest starting with similar plan presented in Table 5, then expanding it to include all days if possible. Try to perform at least 90 to 120 minutes of cardio 4 days a week, with 2 scheduled rest days. Days 6 and day 7 are interchangeable, and the workout duration may vary depending on the circumstances at the time. Sometimes, I will ride 45, 50, or 60 miles if I am preparing for an event, but I normally ride for sixty minutes, 3 to 4 times per week when I am just on "regular cardio maintenance".

Since I cycle, I also have a winter, or home "trainer," plan that is somewhat different than above (Example in Figure 5). It includes three to five days on a trainer at home or on a bike at the gym. This could be another good place to start your cardio plan. A trainer can be a stationary bike or a device that you attach to your bicycle. There are many trainer devices to choose from and the entry level is very affordable. If you do choose a trainer for cardio, make sure that it can easily connect with an app or computer so that you can ride online with others.

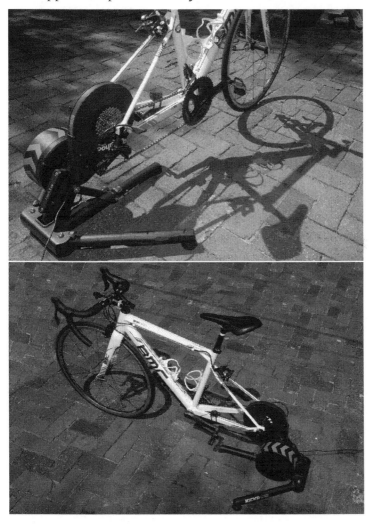

Figure 5. Example of Road bike hooked up to a "Trainer" Setup.

It can be boring sitting on a stationary bike but to make it fun you can ride with others in virtual reality. During my trainer time, I will sometimes watch some sort of educational video. When I have a heavy work schedule, the trainer at home helps me keep with my cardio goals if I cannot get outside.

Day	Zone	Notes on Exercise
Day 1:	Z2/Z3	40 to 80 minutes
Day 2:	Intervals	35 to 55 minutes
Day 3:	Rest Day	
Day 4:	Z2/Z3	40 to 80 minutes
Day 5:	Intervals	35 to 55 minutes
Day 6:	Z2/Z3	40 to 80 minutes
Day 7:	Rest Day	

Table 6 - Base cardio workout schedule for starting and intermediate programs - Home Trainer or Wintertime workouts.

A philosophy to also think about is mixing exercises. It is best to mix cardio and strength workouts to achieve maximum health and performance. Also, remember that it is possible to overuse muscles while working out. We do not want to throw muscle groups out of balance because a certain muscle group has been neglected during our workout scheme. If this happens, you will throw your body into pain as discussed during the mobility section. Next, to complete the whole physical activity picture, we will need to discuss core and strength training.

Cardio training is half the story for a workout plan.

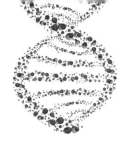

CHAPTER 10:

CORE STRENGTH TRAINING AND GENERAL PHYSICAL ACTIVITY

The conversation now moves from cardio training to improving muscle strength. Core strength training workouts take many forms. While working on mobility aspects, we might want to also start working on core strength exercises. For example, I started with simple push-ups, sit-ups, and other low weight exercises to rebuild my core strength (See Appendix 3 for examples of some of the exercises). Where you start with a core workout plan is dependent on the number of years that you have not been in the gym. When you get back to the gym, make it a competition with yourself. Don't try to compete with those around you. Another suggestion is to work out with someone that is at the same skill level as you.

For this book, my definition of core strength training, in terms of the N-of-1 Challenge, is low-weight, high-rep exercises that will elevate your heart rate while improving muscle strength. I started here because my back and shoulder muscles were so dysfunctional. I had overused some muscles and underused others and found that this type of exercise regimen was the most helpful for balancing my muscles again.

When I started taking control of my health five years ago, I was not going to the gym at all and my back would hurt if I did the wrong exercises or if tried to lift too much weight. I had let my core muscle strength deteriorate since at least 2007 and had severely sprained my wrist in 2011. When I started looking for workouts, a friend suggested some high-intensity interval training videos (HIIT). I started down this path, but it was a bit too much for my knees, so I switched to cycling for my cardio needs. Shortly after that, I found the gym and started a twelve-exercise regimen that I could perform at a faster pace with more reps. I also purchased a set of adjustable dumbbell weights so that I could perform workouts at home. To help save on time because the day can be busy, I suggest purchasing a set of adjustable dumb-bells (Figure 6). My wife and I also purchased me a set of kettlebells (Figure 7). The dumbbell set that I have can be adjusted between 10 to 55 pounds. Sometimes there is not enough time to go to the gym, so it is nice to perform some sort of workout at home before showering for work.

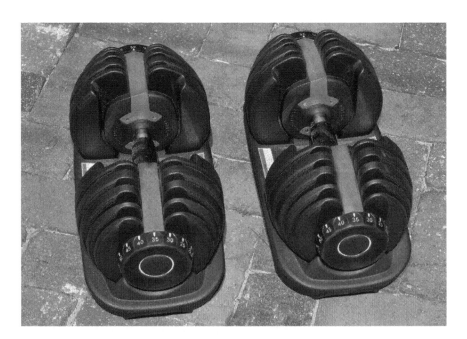

Figure 6. Example of adjustable dumbbells that can be used for quick, at-home training.

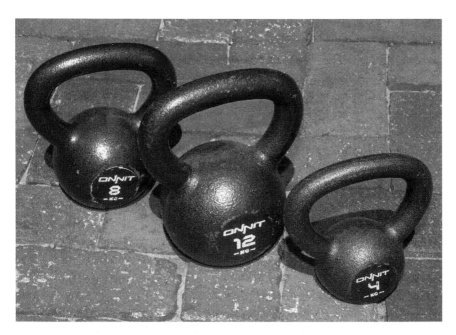

Figure 7. Example of kettlebells that can be used for quick, at-home training.

I have found that it's fun to mix types of exercises. This is great for muscle development and it also keeps the workout fresh and new. I don't typically go into the gym and powerlift because my previous sports injuries and lower back issues do not allow me to do this sort of workout. I go to the gym and lift what I can. I don't need to compete with the guy (or gal) that is bench pressing 250 pounds.

My N-of-1 goal and challenge is to make it to the gym at least three times per week for at least 40 to 60 minutes. This complements my goal of 60 to 100 miles of cardio per week (or three to four bike rides per week). *Key Note: Exercise does not need to be a lengthy process.* Perform fun, meaningful exercise over the course of a 40- to 60-minute workout. If you can keep this up, you will build momentum. If you only have 30 minutes, still perform some sort of exercise. Remember, journaling will help you see the improvements that you reach. At the end of this section, I will re-list the best practices for helping you achieve your goals.

Keep in mind that the goal is to help strengthen your core muscles. One of the most important aspects of core strength training is form. A second important aspect is balancing strength in all of our muscle groups. Learn the proper motion and form for the specific exercise that you perform. It may be tempting to push yourself and increase the amount of weight before you're ready. Don't do it. This isn't about maxing out or proving you can still lift as much as you could in college.

In the end, the beauty of this exercise plan is that it can be 40 to 55 minutes, depending on your scheme and plan. The following is an example of a core strength training program to get you started.

Three or Four Days per Week Basic Core Weight Training

These exercises are designed to mix the muscle groups throughout the course of the week and work to create balance. Again, use lower weight and perform high reps. From the list below, perform three to four sets of each. In Appendix 3 of this book, I provide pictures of example exercises described in this section. This scheme is designed to be quick and to fit into a busy schedule. Remember, the goal is to work out three to four days per week, rotating through these Core Groups:

Core Group 1:	(A) Push-up	(B) Flys
	(C) Bicep Curl	(D) Triceps Curl
	(E) Front Curl	(F) Hammer Curl
	(G) Pull-ups	(H) Sit-ups
Core Group 2:	(I) Lower Back	(J) Squats
	(K) Bench Row	(L) Lat Pulldown
	(M) Standing Row	(N) Shrug
	(O) Shoulder Press	(P) Leg-lift

There are numerous styles of exercise for each of the above listed needs. While performing these exercises (Examples in Appendix 3) you can use body weight, elastic bands (Seen in Figure 3), kettlebells (Figure 7), dumbbells, or visit the gym. There are often gyms that have specific machines setup that can be used for a core workout. In the end, there are numerous resources for finding exercises that you may want to perform but remember that form is one of the most important aspects while performing exercise. If you have questions about form, please visit your local expert for extra coaching.

For me, I performed this type of workout scheme for at least a year before adding more weight to lift. The next section covers more advanced workouts that we can pursue after we have fixed our core strength needs.

Powerlifting for Strength Training

During my twenties, I lifted much more weight and was more into strength training for power. I was more focused on the maximum amount of weight for performance. Then, I missed about ten years of not really working out - there were times when I started to work out again, but my shoulder and back would hurt, so I would eventually stop again. Four years ago, I started to make a consistent effort, learning to work within what my body would let me do. Only recently have I started to add more weight to my workout regimen. I don't powerlift, but now I have increased the number of exercises per workout. For example, I will now perform more than one exercise for each muscle group.

For some people, strength training is what they really enjoy. But if it has been some time since you've worked out, it is best to *not* go right into the gym and lift like you are in your twenties. Powerlifting can be dangerous if you have not been to the gym for many years. All training can be dangerous if you do not know what you are doing - poor form can lead to injury. Unless you have an aptitude for power lifting, I strongly suggest hiring a coach or a trainer for this type of workout.

When it comes to powerlifting, maxing the amount of weight we lift is the goal. Improvements will be based on lifting increased weight overtime. In addition to the variations in exercises and the amount of weight you use, powerlifting will also require you to follow a specific diet, often with supplements, to help build muscle.

For a distinction, when I perform a core workout, I keep the weight the same for each exercise and perform a high number of reps (8 to 12). As I improve in strength, I raise the weight for the particular exercise over time. For a core workout, I don't change the amount of weight during that day for that exercise. The way I look at powerlifting - you start at a lower weight than your max, and as you go through the exercise, the weight is increased per set. Each set has less reps as you go up in weight. The last set for a particular exercise is usually near your maximum amount of weight for a shorter number of reps.

I chose to perform the core workout style because I cannot lift near my max due to a few back injuries that I still have to monitor. I focus on muscle groups and form as opposed to trying to bench press 300 pounds.

If your N-of-1 goal is to bulk up, then power lifting is the route to go. I find that core strength training keeps me exactly where I want to be with my health.

From where I started with the core strength training above, I have added more weight as my body has healed. I also have added more exercises and perform more than one exercise for each muscle group. The above core workout is designed to be performed at home with the adjustable dumbbells I suggested (or at the gym, of course). Since I have been working out for 4 years now and my core strength is much better, I have added some powerlifting concepts to my workout—but bulking up is not my goal.

A typical core strength week now looks like this:

Every Other Day Rotation		
Rotation	Description	Notes
Workout 1	Chest, Arms, and Abs	12 exercises total
Workout 2	Back, Shoulders, Legs and Abs	12 exercises total
Workout 3	Core, Small Muscle Groups, and Abs	12 exercises total
Workout 4	Bonus Day	Gym Rotation or Other Activity

Table 7 - Base core-strength workout - Advancement from Initial Core Strength Training.

The combinations of workouts can be endless! In the end, three of the most important aspects are:

(1) Find someone to work out with to create accountability; this makes the workouts fun and will help you maintain a plan.

(2) A workout can be completed in 45 to 60 minutes and will need a commitment of 3 to 4 days per week. Even if you can only perform a short, 30-minute workout, this will be better than nothing.

(3) Journal! You can't measure improvements without journaling.

Outdoor and Recreational Training

The list of outdoor and recreational training possibilities are endless, but here are some great options that will increase your heart rate or provide some core strength help:

- Road cycling and mountain biking
- Jogging, walking
- Swimming
- Racquetball or tennis
- Kayaking or canoeing
- Backwoods hiking and camping (carrying a backpack)
- Golfing (walking the course, not riding in a golf cart)
- Rock climbing
- Skiing or snowboarding
- Water skiing or other water sports
- Paddle boarding, surfing, and kite sailing
- Boat sailing

The number of outdoor activities available are endless. The most important part of the physical activity you choose: You should enjoy it!

The N-of-1 Challenge Summary for Physical Activities

As with all things in life, the more we do it, the better we get at it. It follows that the more work you put into maintaining a great cardio system, the greater return you see in the long run. The more cardio exercise you commit to, the easier it becomes. On the other hand, if you only perform cardio work once per week, you will see minimal returns, and it won't get any easier.

Gains in strength training can be slow and tedious, especially if you have not been to the gym for many years. For example, I had several weak muscles in my back. I experienced shoulder pain, some spinal issues, knee pain, and a hip flexor issue. Due to my work schedule and lifestyle, I took almost a ten-year break from any real physical activity. Another issue that I had to deal with resulted from sitting too long at desks while writing, reading, performing research, and looking at data.

Over the last four years, I have adjusted my personal physical activities to include and exclude certain exercises. For example, I love tennis, but I can no longer play. From many years of baseball and a partially torn clavicle, it is too painful. As well, I cannot really jog or run. I worked to add it to my plan, but it does increase the amount of pain I live with in my knees, hips, and back. I can still hike up to ten miles in a day and I try to walk at least five to eight miles per week. I have found cycling (on a road bike and at the gym) to be the best form of cardio for me. I get all of the cardio benefits from cycling without the pain. However, cycling does come with risks, as does all exercise. These are just some examples of where my N-of-1 has landed with me with regards to my cardio work.

Attainable Goals (Short and Long-Term)

Your attainable goals (short and long-term) will be dependent on your history and current state of health. Setting your sights too high can be just as detrimental; you can hurt yourself or become discouraged. If there is an unrealistic goal, call it what it is—don't injure yourself. Coaches can be helpful with setting and achieving realistic goals. Set encouraging, realistic goals if you are in a "re-start" phase of your life.

Keep a Fitness Journal

Depending on the physical activities that we choose, we need to record the information. If a month goes by and you only have three or four entries, the plan needs to be revisited. There are several apps and software programs that can be used to journal workouts and collect data such as workout time, heart rate, and many other metrics. One of my favorite apps is STRAVA. In the cardio chapter, I shared and reviewed my number of miles per day cycling journal. Below, **Figure 8** is an example of my workout data from just tracking the number of workouts per month. This does not include the number of bike rides, just the number of core strength workouts per month.

To again show the power of journaling, I generated a graph to show how many days per month I work out. When you journal, you will be able to see trends and you will also be able to track your progress to reach your goals. The change will not be easy in the beginning and it may be difficult to get on track. Just take a look at my data. For the first year, I had a hard time with consistent workouts. However, I did not get discouraged. Now, I consistently reach my monthly goals. Compared to where I started, I can lift much more weight and I have fully evolved my work out plan. I often try to change my scheme every six months now.

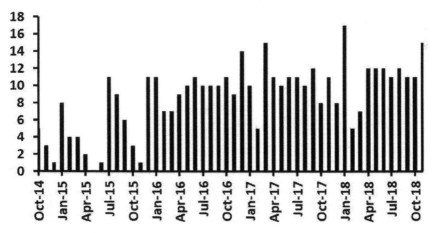

Figure 8 - Number of workouts each month. Note the increase in consistency and note the February 17 counts. I was sick with a cold or flu that month. Other bars, such as Feb/Mar 2018 represent a death in the family and when we moved from Tennessee to Florida.

Accountability Coach

Sometimes, even self-motivated people lose their drive or just get caught up with life. We have to take care of ourselves because no one else is going to. A good coach or specialist will help you plan and reach goals. If you feel that you need a coach or trainer, you should consider hiring one. Family members might not make the best choice for accountability.

For my story, I was able to grow my self-motivation without a trainer. I was able to change my diet and maintain a constant workout schedule because something turned on inside of me. I do have coaches in other areas of my life, but I was able to become aware of what my body was telling me. When searching for leadership, not all coaches and trainers are the same. Some coaches will make better pairs with certain people naturally.

In the end, make sure that you ask or shop around so that you find the best fit for your personality and needs.

Planning Chart for the N-of-1 Challenge

In Chapter 13, I have placed a simple chart to be filled out. This could be considered your first journal entry. The first assessment is to fill out your weekly schedule. Look at where you may pick off time to stretch or workout. The goal is to make time for yourself so that you can achieve new lifestyle and health goals. Start by adding your everyday life items, then find times when workouts can be added. You may need to alter some of your everyday life items to make room for a workout. If I put something on a schedule, I usually worked to achieve it. This can be a great start to changing some "bulk scheduling habits" that we may be un-aware of.

If you are in a "re-start" phase, work to reclaim two hours of your week so that you can work towards a healthy lifestyle.

But once we put the data down on paper, how do we move forward? The next part of this book is on mind-space and offers some suggestions on how to achieve these goals. We now come full circle from the beginning of the book. We started out the discussion on habits and other aspects of mental health management. Now we finish with this concept in the last part of the book.

PART 4:
MIND-SPACE AND MENTAL-HEALTH MANAGEMENT

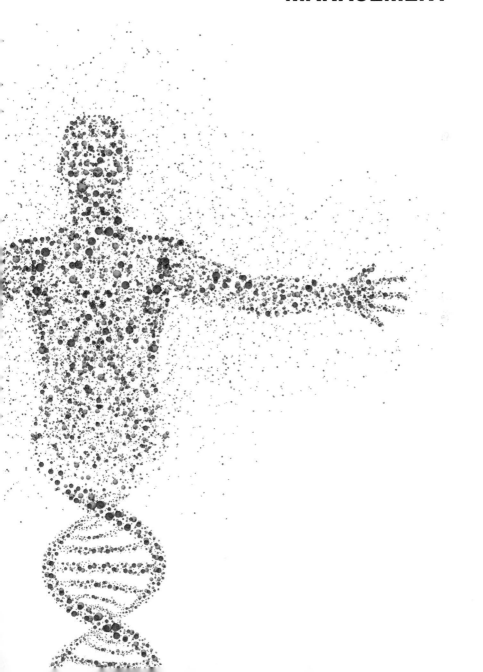

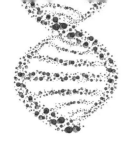

CHAPTER 11:
MIND-SPACE AND MENTAL BURNOUT

As we go through life, we and the people around us change. As we age, our bodies also change. Often, we don't pay attention to these changes, and we just continue with the same habits to manage our lives. It is human nature to continue the same habits, even though we know that we should change at times. However, if we are mindful of our changing environments and make the correct adjustments as we age, we can alleviate unnecessary diseases and pain with proper nutrition and increased physical activities. Parts 2 and 3 of this book discuss the importance of nutrition and core strength, as well as actions we can perform to improve these areas of our lives.

The next piece to discuss is the proper management of our minds and mental health. With management, we can overcome anything in our lives. If your health has slipped, practicing mindfulness will help power you forward. Throughout this book, I have been using the term "mind-space." For the purpose of this discussion, I would like to define mind-space as the total amount of thoughts that one can have (subconscious and conscious). To continue this discussion, let's only consider the conscious or cognitive part of our mind-space, i.e. we are not going to consider the subconscious or dreams.

We only want to consider the mind-space that involves managing our thoughts while we are awake. We want to think about mind-space in a similar mindset as the discussion during the first part of this book - we defined that we are only going to consider the parts of our lives that we can control. With regards to mind-space, some of the concepts that we can control could be relationships with other people, how we view ourselves, and the choices that we make. We can expand upon this list, but most importantly, if we spend time on managing and paying attention to our choices and habits, we can change them.

Let's expand the analogy and describe mind-space as money or finance—something we spend, or a budget. To help, I am working to make a similar analogy to counting calories as found in Chapter 5. Let's assign $1,000 to our own mind-space budget. Next, for discussion, let's subtract $500 for subconscious activities. The numbers are arbitrary but are being used to reach a point. That leaves $500 for the conscious portion of mind-space. The analogy continues to: How much of our mind-space value are we spending on the relationships that we have?

"Overhead" is low when you connect with people that are positive influencers in your life (overhead is a term used in business to describe fixed costs for operations). Overhead is high when you have negative influencers in your life. Let's say overhead for positive influencers is $100, and for negative influencers is $300. With the positive influencers, that leaves $400 of mental-space to spend; whereas negative influencers will leave you with $200. I think you can see where I am going with this. You can apply this logic to all sorts of influences in your life. Everyone has their own mind-space budget to spend on life. Some people have bigger budgets than others, just like some people are natural athletes, and others don't have a sweet tooth.

List out and journal the positive and negative influencers in your life. Use the same journaling concepts described earlier. You can just write your thoughts down in a paperback journal.

In my opinion, mind-space is finite. We all have our own budget that we can spend before we start feeling burnt out or mentally fatigued. Reaching burn out or mental fatigue can be managed by habits. Negative habits cost more or have higher overhead than positive habits. If we are maintaining healthy, positive habits, we have more mind-space to spend on our family, friends, and society in general. We want to manage our mind-space so that we can manage our habits. This is circular logic, but I think this is why we often get trapped in life when we are going in circles with bad habits. In the end, we have to actively manage our life with regards to nutrition and core strength. We can't let our habits control our mind-space.

You can really only do one thing at a time or (logically) think about one thing at a time. Earlier during the book, I referenced *The Power of Now* **(REF 1)** to be a great read because it speaks about how individuals need to focus on what we can do, when we can do it. We need to focus on what we can do now. Our society lives with desire for things we do not have, and we all complain way too much. If we would stop and focus on what is right in front of us and what we need to do, we would all have better lives. If you desire to be healthy, then take the actions needed. If you treat yourself well, you will find that you have more mind-space for improved relationships. Most often, if you are not treating yourself well, then you are probably not doing well. If you are maxed out with your mind-space budget, you will have none to spend on those you love.

Everyone is born with different aptitudes and abilities. Discover and place value on your own aptitude and abilities. Some people have more mind-space to spend on different aptitudes and abilities. Generally speaking, I have found that those with overactive brains have a harder time managing their mind-space at times, but other people have fortitude solid as a rock. For me, I have an easy time maintaining a workout regimen and a specific diet. I think that this may be due to being part of several team sports and generally not having a sweet tooth. However, I have a hard time "turning my brain off" when it comes to working. As mentioned before, I would typically work 50- to 70-hour weeks, with no real time to relax or enjoy certain aspects of life. Over the years, I burnt out with not much energy to give those of importance in my life. When I realized this, I worked to get my workaholic mindset under control.

Some of us simply need to slow down. On the other end, some of us need extra motivation to get to the next level and reach our goals. However, if all you do is "go," this can put you into classical mental burnout. If you are in physical pain from an overuse injury, you will think about that pain. If all you do is work, there will be no time for anything else. If you have strong fortitude and mental-space, you will be able to absorb more of life. You will be able to manage the daily nuances of life and be a light in other's lives.

Place value on your relationships and the other aspects of your life. Place value on the positive and negative influencers in your life. Place values on what you eat and the physical activities you perform. Place value on yourself. Take responsibly for actions.

Life on the Road and the People You Meet

At one point during my career, I stayed in over 400 hotel rooms during a two-year period. I was a top performer covering thirteen states. I was winning. I *owned* my territory.

When I first started this phase of my life, I chose to stay at a certain hotel chain. They were all designed to have the same lobby and design. Mentally, this turned out to be rough for me because there were plenty of times when I woke up and didn't know what city I was in. So, I switched to a different brand that had a different look in the cities I traveled to. This gave me comfort; I tricked myself into believing that I had homes that I would travel to. Often, after visiting several clients in three different cities during a week, I would go to the wrong hotel room; I would go to the room number that I had stayed in the previous night. This mental fragmentation became more frequent as I traveled. In the back of my mind, I started to think that might be a problem, but the front of my mind said it was okay and normal. As my colleagues had told me, I was a true road warrior!

Some people have the mental fortitude to maintain a heavy travel lifestyle. I have met and worked with many of them, and I honestly don't know how they do it. I really love to travel, but not 400 hotel rooms per year.

Traveling is fun, and not just for the professional interactions; I enjoy going to local restaurants to see what's going on in that part of the country. It's a blast. Some of my favorite times were in Dallas, San Francisco, Boston, or Birmingham—just talking with locals at dinner or at the bar to learn about them, what's going on, and their views on the world. I absorbed it all but to a fault. As time went on, it became more of a burden.

One of the reasons that I prepared this book is because of all the stories that I heard from people while traveling. I saw and spoke with many unhealthy, negative people. I also spoke with healthy, positive people, but mostly negative-minded people. An interesting aspect of my travels and life is that most everyone I spoke to told me about their life and problems. Most of them knew what they needed to do to improve their lives but, strangely, they did not want to take the steps needed to fix the problem. Humans love to complain. It's one of our least attractive traits—making excuses to keep our bad habits because of the difficulty of change.

Over a couple of years, I just expected to hear another sob story or some sort of negative accusation of some absurdity. Everyone wanted to tell a story, but many people did not want to take control of their lives or health. Everyone just wanted to complain about their life! Humans excel at complaining and making problems where they don't exist. Nutrition and physical activity are perfect examples of how humans lie to themselves. It's how we get to become unhealthy—ignoring the truth of our basic need for good nutrition and physical activity. We continue to move through time, and the excuses go on and on. Then BAM! Obesity, pre-diabetes, Type 2 diabetes, elevated cholesterol, a heart attack, double bypass surgery, etc. Most health problems stem from years of overuse, neglect, and lying to ourselves.

In the end, I really enjoy traveling and learning about people's passions. However, I found that most people are not focused on their passion; they are focused on their pain. They just want to talk about what's wrong, not what's right about the world. I would never have thought that I would allow myself to be burdened by all these stories. I was disappointed that people preferred to complain about their situations than actually try to do something to fix them.

Of course, working stressful, 70-hour weeks does not lead to happiness. My priorities had to change, and I needed a break. I was living my own hypocrisy, but I had become aware in many ways. I had started my nutrition and core strength recovery about one year before my full mental burnout. At the time, I was making minimal gains in losing weight and strength training. This is because I did not work on mind-space until I had reached mental burnout. It was my blind- spot. I literally woke up one day and could not get the engine to start.

I am not sure what your stress points are or where you are in terms of your mind-space "budget." Only you know for sure. For me, I was a workaholic and a weekend warrior. I was pushing myself too hard and needed to slow down. I did not sleep. But since my "crash," I have adopted different management schemes for the various areas of my life. One of the concepts that I have known about is the mind-body connection or understanding what your body is telling you.

The Mind-Body Connection

Many of the people I spoke with while preparing this book were able to start improving their health when they made a connection between how they feel and how they treat themselves. They made a mind-body connection with their nutrition and physical activity.

Many of us don't even know that we can feel better. We have lived certain lifestyles for numerous years while being blind to the chronic addition of weight because of poor diet and lack of physical activity. It is easy to understand what feeling sick means when you get something like a bad cold or flu. You get sick for a week, the cough lingers for a week or two, then you finally feel better. There is a noticeable difference—the process of getting the flu and healing. But with obesity and chronic illness, we don't seem to make the same mental connection. We will not get better or lose weight unless we put in an effort. Healing from the common cold is not about effort; it just takes time.

Obesity arrives after years of progressive neglect. It's not the same as having a cold or flu for a week. It can be hard to understand a progressive disease because you simply don't notice it as it creeps up on you. If your mind is not connected to your body, you might not be paying attention. You are just continuing to live with the same bad habits that are considered good rationalizations.

During my research for the book, I came across a short book called *Mind-Body Connection Therapies* by Merrily A. Kuhn, RN, Ph.D. Here are some quotes from the book that I found to be within the same spirit of what we are discussing **(REF 35)**.

"The idea that a person can learn to modify his or her own vital functions is relatively new. Before the 1960s, most scientists believed that autonomic functions such as heart rate and pulse, digestion, blood pressure, brain waves, and muscle behavior, could not be voluntarily controlled. Recently, biofeedback, along with other methods of self-regulation, such as guided imagery, progressive relaxation, and meditation, has found widespread acceptance among physiologist and psychologist alike."

"The chemicals we put in our body change the internal equilibrium. Thus, when we get external stimuli, we are no longer able to maintain a health equilibrium."

"... we spend almost nothing to treat the cause of chronic disease before major illness develops."

"These examples are illustrations of the body's natural tendency towards repairing itself. This tendency is known as homeostasis, the maintenance of the body's internal organs and defenses to compensate for external health hazards... symptoms should be left alone so that the repair process can take place."

The main point of this discussion is that you can connect your mind with your body. You can draw a connection between what you put in your body and how you feel. The chemicals that you put in your body (or food) will have a direct effect on you. In the end, there are several paths to reaching a mind-body connection. There are many practices that one can use to help manage mind-space.

To review, in a similar sense to nutrition and physical activity journaling, sit down and write out the positive and negative influences in your life. Once you have defined what these influences are, you can start to make changes. Just like nutrition and physical activity, there are several different paths to managing mind-space. One particular type of management would be meditation.

For the rest of this book, I will focus on mind-space management through meditation, the practice of yoga, and prayer.

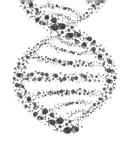

CHAPTER 12:

MEDITATION, THE PRACTICE OF YOGA, AND PRAYER

Meditation can take many forms, but it is fundamentally the art of "obtaining relaxation through mental practice." The two major forms of meditation can be described as concentrative and mindfulness. During concentrative meditation, your mind focuses on a sound, your breathing, or an image. With mindfulness meditation, you focus on the awareness of feelings, images, thoughts, sounds, and smells that pass through the mind *without* concentrating on them; you simply observe them. The goal of such mindfulness is to gain a nonreactive, clear, calmer state of being.

I found concentrative meditation to be easier to start with, rather than mindfulness meditation. My breakthrough in meditation came from using a phone app to help with guided meditations. I could not get into a meditative state without a guide. The effect of this guide is the same as a weight training coach. I need a coach to help with meditative practices.

Meditation has been helpful for my personal needs and may help you with mind-space management. Remember, one of my goals with this book is to present different practices that may help you improve your health. Not only is yoga a great way to practice meditation, it helps with mobility and physical activity. I feel incredibly exhausted and mentally relieved after a good session. Yoga has many forms and has several benefits for mind-space and overall health. Could this be a practice for your N-of-1 Challenge and goals?

Yoga for Mind-Space Management and Health

Yoga can be considered one of the oldest forms of healthcare practices in the world. Over the centuries, many different forms have been created by new yoga masters for different benefits. Until I researched yoga and started to practice, I did not know that there were so many forms. As well, all of the instructors are different in the forms and classes they teach. I started yoga less than a year ago and have found the benefits of yoga to be very helpful. I am not an expert or an authority on yoga, but it has opened me to another great tool that has helped me improve both mobility and manage mind-space.

There are different forms of yoga and it's best to perform research on what type you would like to work on. When I started yoga, it kicked my butt—even with my current workout and cardio regimen. I was sore for three days because I had activated certain deep core muscle groups. My practice has greatly improved since I started. Practicing yoga can help with three key aspects of health: mobility, core strength, and mind-space.

There are several excellent sources of information for yoga and the different forms on the internet. Below are the main forms of yoga and some base information to help you understand the difference between the forms. Generally, yoga studios suggest that you start with a form and go for at least three sessions before deciding.

Hatha Yoga

All physical yoga practice is considered Hatha Yoga. Literally, Hatha means 'force' and is traditionally defined as 'the yoga of force', or 'the means of attaining a state of yoga through force'. You can also interpret Hatha to mean physical postures, not a specific style. A third meaning for Hatha includes the concept of balancing the sun and the moon or the lunar and the solar energies in the body. With a simple Hatha class, most of the time, you're just cycling through postures. There is often no linking the positions together. As opposed to other forms of yoga, the sequence could come together and that makes sense (i.e. activation of certain muscle groups in order), or it could make no sense at all.

Ashtanga and Vinyasa Yoga

Sri K. Pattabhi Jois and T. Krishnamacharya started these forms of yoga during the 20th century. Ashtanga and Vinyasa Yoga both simply mean the practice of connecting breath and movement together. Both of these practices have the same postures during a series; however, Ashtanga is going to be a set series and Vinyasa is going to be a free flow session. Another way to look at it, Vinyasa Yoga is a derivative of Ashtanga Yoga. Both are is also known as "power yoga," as there is dynamic energy that goes into the practice of this form.

I primarily work with Ashtanga Yoga because it has a set series. When I perform yoga during the morning, the set series helps me add structure to my day.

Iyengar Yoga

Iyengar yoga is form that has very specific alignments and postures. A typical session will include maybe five positions over and over again during the sequence in increments. During the sessions, one will not go to a fullest expression. This means that rather than jumping straight to the yoga postures found in Ashtanga and Vinyasa Yoga, Iyengar teaches you how to get there. Interestingly, during my research, I found several sources that suggested that the postures we see today came into existence over the last 50 years.

The diversity of yoga forms arises from student-teacher interactions. For example, Iyengar was a student of Krishnamacharya, who can be considered the "grandfather" of Ashtanga Yoga. Iyengar branched off and started his own practice because he was essentially injured by following Krishnamacharya teachings and practice. Iyengar felt that Krishnamacharya's practice was a bit too aggressive and difficult. Thus, he slowed the movements down and developed more of a therapeutic approach. In the end, Iyengar's sequences are designed for improved health and in one of his books, he has specific sequences for certain illnesses—asthma, depression, high blood pressure, or diabetes. I have not personally tried this form of yoga. I really enjoy the set Ashtanga "Power" Yoga with a set series.

Bikram Yoga

Bikram Choudhury was a student of Krishna Matera from the Ashtanga lineage who broke off from the mainstream. Bikram Yoga is a set series of 26 postures and is taught in a hot room. This is what is often referred to as "hot yoga" — the sequences are performed at 105 degrees Fahrenheit. He started hot yoga and others came along and modified the postures. In this practice; we simply move from one posture to another posture (26 in total), holding each posture twice. This is primarily called 'Hot Yoga' now.

Kundalini Yoga

Kundalini yoga is about moving the Shiva Shakti energy within us and raising that vibration throughout the body (or holding on to using the Kundalini energy to bring it out). There are a lot of movements with mantras involved. It is not power yoga like the other forms described earlier. Also this form is very different from Iyengar Yoga. With this type of yoga, you are trying to reach for the energy inside and pull it out. It is considered to be incredibly powerful for releasing positive energy. Those that practice this form claim that they are able to feel the Shiva Shakti energy from the base of the spine and move it around. This is also considered an advanced form and it does take time to reach this level of yoga.

Yin Yoga

Yin Yoga can be considered the "other practice" of yoga. Ashtanga and Vinyasa are "Yang" practices. With yang practices, you're flowing and in constant movement all the time. With the "Yin" practice, you are doing the opposite — you are slowing the movements down. Also, the names of the postures are different than the other styles of yoga. The Yin form of yoga has been around for thousands of years, with debate on when it was first practiced. With a traditional Yin practice, no props are used, and the individual does not go through flows. One might perform 7 postures during an hour session. The goal is to hold postures for anywhere between 3 to 5 minutes. If you are performing traditional Yin, you are not pulling yourself into the posture by letting gravity do the work. The focal point of this practice is to get deep into the layers of connective tissue beyond the muscles—more towards tendons and ligaments in joints in those areas—to open up and make more space.

Final notes on the practice of Yoga as a whole

Over the years, yoga has developed to have several different forms. The different forms arose out of student-teacher relationships and innovation. However, yoga can be considered to be one of the world's oldest forms of healthcare. Outside of the United States, yoga is practiced by both men and women. It is not just a feminine activity, as it is treated in the United States. Could yoga be a practice that helps you with core strength *and* mind-space?

After working through different forms of yoga and instructors, I typically go to Ashtanga Yoga sessions. I like this form of yoga because it has set postures to work through. This set series is something that I try to do every morning, which helps add some physical and mental structure and balance. I also like this form of yoga because it is logical to me. The progression is designed to activate and stretch muscles in a certain order.

If yoga and/or meditation are not for you, there are other options. Yoga and meditation are closely tied to Eastern philosophies. Of course, Western philosophies and prayer can be used to manage mind-space as well. Perhaps you can use yoga for added physical activity on top of prayer and other community activities?

Prayer and Community to Help Manage Mind-Space

We are all mentally wired for community and gathering. We often rely on our community or closest circle to help us get through tough times. For this part of the book, I interviewed Reverend Alfonso Woods to discuss the importance of community, taking care of each other, and prayer. This interview demonstrates how important community is for helping each other through normal everyday situations. How we manage everyday situations is the key to maintaining mental health. If we let every little thing get us down, how can we live a fulfilling life?

When we struggle, we need to know that there is someone there to support us. In the interview, we see how important community is for the success of individuals and how supporting each other can lead to improved results. As part of your N-of-1 Challenge, you may need to find a new support system or new friends who have similar interests. You also may need to find something bigger to believe in so that you don't focus solely on your own problems.

Reverend A. Woods on Prayer and Community

Many people, specifically in the stories part of this book, state that they needed a support group or a coach when trying to reach their goals for improving their health. I'm curious about community and support from your perspective—in terms of prayer and community.

I'll be happy to answer that. I'm 62 years old, and I've been a part of a community of faith since I was 16. I actually remember the day that I joined the church. Our family was very much about faith. The community for us was our extended church family.

That said, not everybody lends themselves to being trusting and buddy-buddy with a lot of other people. Some people are just loners. They're more comfortable by themselves, away from a lot of other people. But what I have witnessed is that from a holistic health standpoint—physical, mental, and spiritual—people tend to fare a whole lot better in a community. I don't necessarily mean a community where people are with each other every day, in and out, doing everything together. I mean an environment where they can find support when they need it or can give support when others needed it.

There is a small, close-knit community, usually including close family members. Then there's a broader community, which could be a group of people who share the same interests as you. They socialize together. In my case, it tends to be people who share the same faith—we share our same beliefs in the same trust.

Now that I am a pastor, what I have found is that people who attend church services—and on a regular basis—come because they bring something with them and take something away from the experience. We all have the need for a loving, caring, supportive environment. To be able to hear simple things like, "How are you doing today?", "How's life for you?", "Can I pray for you?", "Can you pray with me?"

When they come into a community of faith, they hear an uplifting word, the promises from God through His word. They also experience witnessing other people who have overcome hardships. They say, "Wow, Joe was really down the other day, but something happened in his life. I can see the change, and I want some of that. I want to feel good." I think that encouragement is important amidst the daily irritations of life.

There's nothing new under the sun. The same challenge that you had yesterday, I probably am having today or will have tomorrow. And you got through it. I can look at that with confidence and be encouraged, trusting that this will pass. Faith is all about believing in the promises of a power far beyond your strength.

Sometimes, it just isn't a great day. But that's not an everyday thing. Community involves helping others and witnessing the power of God in people's lives.

This might sound strange to some people—but if it had not happened to me, I might be suspicious. Once, during worship on a Sunday, I was almost finished with the sermon. I sat down, and there was a spirit that came over me that said, "Somebody needs prayer. Somebody wants to be prayed for." In the end, it actually revealed to me who that person was.

Now, I had not really had any real contact with this person. I didn't really know them very well, and they didn't really attend on a regular basis. That day, they were there assisting somebody else. There was no reason for me to think that this person needed prayer or wanted to be prayed for. I almost just sat down because you don't want to be embarrassed (or to embarrass someone else). But I was obedient. I got up and said, "Before we dismiss, the spirit is telling me that someone needs my prayer. And if that is you, come forward."

Any number of people could have come forward at this point. But the validation was that the person who was revealed in my spirit was the first person to get up. And they got up in a hurry and came up to the front for prayer.

That's where community comes in. If the community hadn't been there, and if the community hadn't been in tune with the goodness of the Universe—the goodness of God—then we as a church would have missed the opportunity to surround this person with support.

It's important to think of yourself, but it's not good to walk around with your burdens all alone. Part of a healthy mind is being able to talk to somebody and share how you are feeling. Because that person may have a perspective that is not encumbered by all of the stuff you're seeing and feeling. They may even give you some helpful direction.

So, you say, "What? I didn't think about that. Thank you. I'm going to take that advice." In many cases, I have done that. I've been better off because now I can approach the problem or the irritation in a healthy way. It could just be an issue that I have with somebody—I'm tired of dealing with this person because they're not doing the right thing or whatever. And somebody else comes in and says, "Why not think about it like this?"

In my book, I interviewed different individuals in patient care. I think that you provide a sort of care for people as a reverend—probably in one of the most important aspects of life. How do you "keep your cup full"? How do you personally deal with the nuances of life?

That is an interesting question because I think you need to determine what the baseline of your mental health is. I might think that I'm doing well, but my baseline is way off. I believe I am functioning pretty well in terms of my mental capacity and my own well-being, but it's a struggle. We battle against the daily irritations of life.

I have a number of things that contribute to the balance that I believe that I have. First off, I'm a happy person. I don't live in a vacuum of sadness or pessimism. I always see the glass as half full. And with that perspective, whatever comes my way, I embrace it as a challenge that is going to leave me more enlightened at the end of the day. So, I'm operating in a realm of positive energy. I came from a very loving and secure family. My father was a hard worker and my mom was a loving parent. They instilled these values in my heart that have followed me to this day.

Growing up, my family went through difficulties, but I never knew that as a child. It was just life. We were poor, but I never knew we were poor. We were a family deeply rooted in faith. I saw my father pray. I saw my mother pray. I saw them deal with tragedy together. I didn't see them shake or become scattered or broken. They attributed their strength to their faith and their trust in God. That has followed me. I have a good relationship with my family, and my immediate family is my wife. We have to be on the same page. We don't always agree, but we don't become disagreeable.

For my own well-being, it helps to have supportive people around me. It helps to know that there are people I can trust. For me, it's important to have a cause beyond the self so that when I get up every day and move into my world of work, I'm not moving because of something I want. I'm actually operating because I believe it's my calling in this world to be a blessing to others. There's always purpose beyond the self. It keeps me from being narcissistic or constantly turning inward.

I know that where I am is just a temporary space. I don't fret about life and death. Like anybody, I want to live a long life. But if my life is going to be long, I want it to be fruitful. I want to be remembered for something and to leave a legacy—a footprint that will last. I want people to say when I'm gone, "He did something. His word could be trusted. If he promised to do something, he would fulfill his promise." And I want people to see in me the goodness that they want to see.

The goodness that people want to see.

For example, I was having breakfast one day with a friend when a guy walked by and said, "Can you spare a dollar? I'm hungry." Why not just buy him breakfast? And so, we did that. And strangely enough, I saw him just yesterday, walking on the street. He thanked me and I was glad to help. That's uplifting to me, being in the position to actually help people. It's those kinds of things that keep me healthy in terms of my mental well-being.

To change directions a bit, I also like to read. I like to expand my mind. I like to think — I watch too much news, but my faith obviously keeps me anchored. From a physical standpoint, I think I could do better. I think my biggest challenge is exercise. I don't work out although, I should. I try not to sit in the office all day. I'll take a walk at least once, maybe twice a day. I try and get in 3,000 steps, to get outside in the fresh air. I try and make healthier choices—not necessarily the healthiest all the time, but I try and make healthier choices. For example, drinking water rather than soda. But I still have a sweet tooth, so I eat a piece of cake or a piece of pie every once in a while.

That leads nicely into the next question. What is your practical diet?

My mom would bake cakes and pies when I was growing up, but it wasn't as though we ate a ton of sweets all the time. What I remember, in terms of eating, was a lot of beans and fresh vegetables. Very rarely did we eat canned vegetables. My father had a garden. So, we would eat squash, potatoes—whatever he was growing. But there were some things that weren't so healthy, like fried chicken. That was a staple. But not a lot of processed food.

We didn't have fast food restaurants in our neighborhood, so we had home-cooked meals almost every day. Most of the time, it involved fresh vegetables. These were vegetables that were either grown or purchased.

As for my practical diet now, I don't have a set regimen in terms of what I eat, but I try to always have fresh veggies like fresh broccoli, corn, and cauliflower. Sometimes it's just a salad. Lately, I've been trying to eat salad without dressing and just enjoy the freshness of the veggies. I don't want iceberg lettuce; it does not have any nutritional value. Give me some mixed greens. I'll chew on some spinach or kale.

My wife and I don't make a habit of preparing canned veggies. We eat most vegetables. Since I cook them, it's nothing for me to stop in a supermarket on the way home and grab this or that. We cook fried chicken. Or we might buy a roasted chicken.

My wife and I have red meat maybe twice per month. Does that sound kind of similar? We eat mostly chicken and fish, sometimes pork.

My wife might buy some pork steaks. It's called "the other white meat." So, that might be on a dinner plate. We love fish. We love seafood. I try and buy fresh seafood sometimes right from the fishermen.

Where do you get your primary carbohydrates from?

We primarily eat wild rice or brown rice. Not a lot of white rice. I did when I was growing up, but that was a staple. We both like potatoes; it's not uncommon for us to have sweet potatoes. Unfortunately, I still love bread.

I don't think that's a bad thing. Too much refined bread is a bad thing.

If I purchase bread, it's a whole grain bread. It's all right to have whole wheat or whole grain. I don't have any problems with gluten intolerance or any wheat allergies. I don't consume much dairy. I have cheese sometimes on a sandwich or maybe cheese on a salad.

I would say 75% of what we eat is fresh vegetables, and my wife drinks a ton of water. I drink more water now than I used to, but normally, I like to have fresh smoothies.

With that, I wanted to touch on something that was very influential during my life. There was a change in my thinking when I went to college. All my life, I have loved to cook. I started working in the cafeteria at Eckerd College.

One of the great things about Eckerd College is that they are at the forefront of bold new directions. They were all about a vegetarian diet add when I was there. They created a program to address the growing number of students who wanted a healthier diet. I ended up being the one who cooked for that program. I cooked lunch and dinner. I was introduced to whole grains, nuts and fruit, honey, meatless casseroles, and brewer's yeast. I started to eat the same foods when I went home; for a while, I didn't eat any meat. My mom couldn't understand it. That has influenced my thinking, and that was back in 1975.

I don't think that was mainstream thinking, or even really thought about back in the 70s. That was definitely cutting-edge thinking based on all of the other information that was out there.

Exactly. They had a special dining room for folks who did not want to eat meat. And we had a whole meal list— healthy food plan—for those who desired that sort of diet. I was responsible for preparing the meals. I started training with a guy named Astore; I was his sous chef. He trained me and ultimately, I began to set up and cook my own meals. It was really great. I began working with honey and nuts and whole grains and yogurt, and that experience carried over to what I do now. So, to get back to your question about steak, we do eat red meat now, but I haven't really been a red meat craver probably since the late 70s.

To me, a steak is a special meal now. That's the way we treat it. I do crave red meat and steaks so when I do, I listen to my body and have a delicious hamburger or a nice big steak.

On one of the topics of this book, we definitely try to stay away from processed sugar as much as possible. We have candy and desserts, but they are not a big part of our diet. I might even get a donut or something every now and then, but it is not the norm. Everything in moderation.

To finish off, I think that's the biggest challenge—managing what the mind tells us. I'll have a great dinner, and there's something my mind says to me, "You need some sweets." So, I'll want a piece of pie or a piece of cake and I don't think there is anything wrong with that. I just think it's a healthier choice not to have dessert all the time.

Perhaps a sense of community is something that you need to add to your N-of-1 Challenge? Do you feel that you need to find people that have something in common? If so, try to find some like-minded people. There are people in your community who enjoy doing the same things you do. If you find people who are like-minded or have similar goals as you, the journey is much easier. Only you can decide if this is something you need.

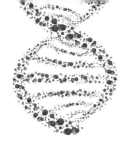

CHAPTER 13:
BRINGING ALL OF THE CONCEPTS TOGETHER

This book has been designed to help bring together basic information about lifestyle changes in three basics concepts for optimal health: nutrition, physical activity, and mind-space management.

We have learned the importance of avoiding obesity and the habits associated with becoming obese. We have also learned the importance of mitigating or (ideally) avoiding overuse injuries associated with these three areas. We have listed some best practices to help improve our health. Probably the most important practice to follow is keeping electronic (or written) journals on what we eat, what we do, and other influences in our lives. We need to pay attention to what we are doing and consuming; it is essential for maintaining a healthy lifestyle.

Much of where I am today is related to my work with Dr. Dex Alvarez, who was my chiropractor back when I was at my lowest heath point. He helped me remember what I needed to do to become healthy again and to get out of my slump. For this book, I went back to Dex and interviewed him about all three aspects of health. Now that we have defined the important aspects, we need to put it all together.

Dex is a chiropractor, but he looks at the whole patient during treatment. Not only does Dex look at the Central Nervous System (CNS), he works on nutrition and habit-forming behaviors. In my opinion, Dex represents a growing class of practitioners—those that can look at each patient holistically, thus finding and fixing the underlying problem for that particular individual.

The following section is the dialogue that we had in regard to his chiropractic practice, some of his own personal practices, and suggestions that many of us can use to improve our lifestyle and health.

Dr. Dex Alvarez Interview and helping to put the Full Message Together

Can you please describe your expertise? Also, what excites you most about practicing and sharing your expertise with others?

I would consider my expertise along the lines of optimizing someone's central nervous system. As a chiropractor by trade, I think the perception is that we are bone crackers or just joint- related specialists. My background is more in neurology— being able to affect a patient's neurology in a positive way to either upregulate certain parts of their central nervous system or alleviate pressure to allow the central nervous system to work optimally. My goal is for a patient to reach the top health they are looking for.

Your brain is the main circuit board. It has to be able to communicate with all of your cells, tissues, and organs. If not, the brain will not be able to coordinate its functions. In order for the full circuit board to work, we need to be able to eliminate a blockage in the CNS that may be creating problems.

I take a look at the biomechanics behind why someone's CNS may not be functioning properly, whether it's from pressure being placed on a part of the brain stem—or part of the actual spinal cord—or from an existing nerve root from a misalignment of a joint or an area of the spine. That spinal joint can cause a degree of inflammation. Or, there may be a lack of mobility in an area that we need to start to correct so that we can again have an optimal flow of information.

In 1972, a Harvard Medical Researcher found that it only took the pressure of a dime on any nerve in your body to cut off the ability to function by 50%. If you think about it, you can put a dime on the back of your hand and in a couple of seconds, you don't even know it's there. But that's enough pressure on, say, your C-7 T-4 nerve that plugs directly into your heart and lungs, to have a decrease of that flow of information by 50%.

Now, that impulse of information from your brain out to that organ is not going to be 100%; let's say it is only about 50% of the needed pulse. Is that heart organ, or your lungs, functioning at 100% at that point? There's no way. They're just not able to communicate because the flow of information is lost. I don't know if I would consider myself an expert in this, but I think I'm very knowledgeable at being able to detect where that impingement is coming from, correct it, and then allow for that function to be regained at 100%. That is my goal with all of my patients.

That's what really excites me; the hunt to try and figure out—what is the true nature of someone's ailment? Are they coming to me because their back hurts or are they coming to me because they can't play with their kids because their back hurts? Or in addition to their back hurting, have they been constipated for years? Some people come to me who can only go to the bathroom a couple of times per week.

So, I look at what the true nature of the problem is. I think that's where it excites me to work with every patient because I get to work backward; I get to figure out the true nature of the problem and what this person really trying to tell me. I want to get down to their emotional level and find out why they came into my office.

This was like the hip flexor event I had. I was in chronic pain for many years. I thought it was my shoulder, but it was really my hip. You worked on me and found the true problem. When it went back into place, the muscle went into spasm. It took me six months for the muscle spasm to go away. It was a cascade issue from my hip being slightly out of place for years!

Right. We could have worked on that muscle until the cows came home, but if we hadn't alleviated the pressure from that joint or nerve, that muscle (and that nerve) would have continued to be constantly aggravated. This caused the muscles to constantly be activated, which was then pulling your hip. We had to work backward to release the pressure on the nerve to allow the muscles to do what they were supposed to do. Then we had to start rehabbing the muscle and retraining it.

Only 10% of your nerve's job is sensory. It's the same nerve system that creates your sciatic nerve—there are five main nerves. There is also a functional

aspect. Nerves plug into your digestive system. They plug into your repro-
ductive organs. They plug into your bladder. Your sinus congestion can be
an upper cervical issue—the upper part of your neck near the base of your
skull. Those are the nerves that feed information to your sinuses behind your
eyes. I can go on for hours about how different parts of your nervous system
affect your bodily functions.

Another thing to think about: By unlocking your vertebrae and allowing
for that proper nervous system flow, allergies will get better. An upper cervical adjustment can increase your immune response by up to 75%. There
is research that shows that specific chiropractic adjustments are the best
way to improve neurological transmission. It has been studied several times,
and the results show that this is the best way to improve the CNS and bodily
functions.

I don't want to solely harp on the nervous system. To me, that is one of
the more important areas, but again that's more of my focus. I don't want
to downplay the importance of nutrition because that's also a tremendous
part of health. For example, there are more neurotransmitters in your gut
than in your brain. So proper gut health, proper nutrition, is tremendous and
important for moving forward in your health.

All of these different systems play a huge role in health—mobility, CNS,
and nutrition. The other aspect that I really like about your book is that you're
also factoring in mindset. This is where I actually start when I see a patient.

**Let's go full circle to the beginning. Let's talk about mindset and how
you manage this with patients.**

It really is all about mindset. I can lead anyone to the water, but they have
to be the one to take the drink. Before I even tackle the central nervous system, I have to work on mindset. Why is your body out of control or in pain?
The first step is to understand that there is no silver bullet to help one get
better. I really wish there were because that would make our jobs a heck of
a lot easier.

**Well, I will say that I've been through probably four or five
chiropractors and you are the first one that started with mindset. It's
a great foundation. As part of your practice, how much is dedicated**

to education? How much do you educate your patients on the central nervous system and nutrition?

Nutrition is a huge part of my practice. On many different levels and for many reasons. The goal is to decrease inflammation. In my opinion, in the United States, this is one of the biggest problems we are dealing with—high levels of inflammation from poor nutrition and CNS injuries. For example, we can link autoimmunity (a problem with inflammation) to rheumatological disorders. We really need to get someone on the proper nutritional path while working on them. We are often successful with education on nutrition while working on the CNS.

Often, we have our patients fill out a three-day diet log and nutritional evaluation. We make that a big topic of conversation. We go through what the patient has been eating, how they're eating, when they're eating, and where they need to adjust. I also discuss supplements when we need to fill in gaps in diet.

Nutrition is something that I talk about with patients every time they're here. Especially after we get to see that nutritional evaluation. Sugar is a monster epidemic and we need to know it as a society. We really need to take a step back and look at how much we're overusing refined sugar. Not to say that all sugars are bad, because, yourself as a biochemist by trade, you know we need glucose.

Initially, we really try to focus on getting our patients off sugar — then we start moving towards the direction of more green, leafy vegetables — farm-raised organic proteins, wild-caught fish. Often, we are working in foods that are high in antioxidants and good fats. We are also fat deprived here in the United States. We need healthy fats in the form of omega-3 and omega-6 and some omega-9. Right now, food is being delivered after being modified. This is also why we look to supplements. It's more difficult to get proper levels of nutrition solely from food.

In the end, a conversation on sugar and carbohydrates is still my jumping-off point with every patient.

For this book, I have been asking about personal nutrition. What is your personal, practical diet?

I think that's a great question because when I talk about nutrition with patients, I try to relay to them that we have to get our bodies back to a point where it can withstand cheesecake, beer, and chicken wings. I say that because my big vice is eating pounds of chicken wings.

For a segue, I performed a hard-core elimination diet for two months. Once I did this, I was able to re-introduce other fun foods into my diet. I did the zero exceptions plan—or what we call our advanced plan diet—that is very heavy in green, leafy vegetables, free range chicken and eggs, wild-caught fish, solely grass-fed beef, zero empty carbohydrates, zero added sugar foods. My energy level went through the roof. My skin cleared up. It was a huge change for me. After eight weeks, I started to allow in more carbohydrates. I'm Spanish, Cuban, and Italian. I love pasta. I love rice. I love sandwiches. So, I started using more grain-related or whole foods.

Now, I eat extremely clean Monday to Friday, but Saturday or Sunday I'm going to drink some beer and eat my body weight in chicken wings. That is what my practical diet is now.

A theme I've found while speaking with different experts is about overuse or underuse injuries. I see sugar consumption as an overuse injury to our biological systems, just like you may see an overuse injury in your patients' CNS or muscle group. Can you speak about overuse in terms of what you see in your practice?

Typically, when I see overuse injuries in my practice, it's overuse related to physical activity or underuse where a patient is deconditioned. This can lead to instability in the spine or joint, which can cause its own issues.

Mental stress and being a workaholic are what finally drove me to make a lifestyle change. My stress hormones were out of control. I remember feeling like I was on an adrenaline rush all the time when I was a road warrior.

Adrenal fatigue is a big one. It affects everybody. Adrenal overuse can be from long periods of stress. Your adrenal glands sitting above your kidneys secrete cortisol, and cortisol in excess can be one of the worst hormones that your body can create. Interestingly, it is known to cause fat retention and a depressed mood. Overuse in that regard is a big one that we see. This often happens with professionals and even people who are not in high-stress professions.

What we really need to do is work on managing stress. How do we alle-viate that stress? Then we might start toning exercise down to a moderate run, rather than an extreme run, to try to get rid of all the stress. Then we can take physical stressors off. So again, working backward being investigative and trying to figure out the true root of someone's problem.

You work in the field of patient care, and you see many patients who are possibly in their worst pain. How do *you* "fill your cup," so to speak, and maintain your own personal mind-space?

That was a struggle, especially during the beginning of my practice. How was I supposed to absorb all this energy and care for these patients and myself?

When patients are coming in and unloading all of this pain, suffering, and frustration, it really affected me quite a bit at the beginning. I had to find ways to practice what I preached to deal with all the energy. I spoke with practice management coaches, other doctors, people that had been in the field longer than I have. I wanted to find out how they dealt with it. In the end, they told me I had to find my own kind of mental release.

That is another theme in the book. We all need to find our own path to health. We all have our own N-of-1 Challenge to meet.

Now, I meditate every day. I especially meditate during the mornings. I also perform self-affirmation during this time. I just try to remind myself of how lucky and blessed I am to be able to solve these problems—to be able to be given the challenges that I'm given every day and help the people I've seen. That alone helps me out tremendously. I try to come up with at least five things I'm thankful for in the morning, then, every night when I go to sleep, five things that I learned that I was thankful for during that day. That simple exercise helped me mentally to have a physical release.

Being active is a huge part of my life. I was an athlete my whole life, but when you start having a family, a business, a practice, it drains your personal time. What I am talking about is carving out a schedule. You have to schedule maintenance for yourself.

I wake up every morning at 5:00 a.m. and take a shower. I don't speak at any point during that time. I try to stay silent and stay in my head and go through a meditative state while I'm exercising. Then I get into the office, and I try to remain silent for as long as possible. I really don't say too much until my staff comes in at 7:00 a.m.

Also, I fish. This taught me patience. That was a big thing for me. I'm very high energy. I've been that way since I was a kid, and my dad told me one time that I don't handle stress well. As a med student, in chiropractic school, he taught me that. When I hear something like that, I take it as a challenge. I had to figure out a way to be able to manage stress better. Fishing taught me to be able to let my mind release and concentrate on something that's out of my control. And that has helped me out tremendously. My wife will tell you that if I don't go fishing at least once per week, I'm an ornery person.

It's just those little things for me—finding a way to have a mental release and understanding that no matter how hard life gets or how stressful things can become, there's so much to be thankful for.

In the end, you have to put in the work, because no one else is going to do it for you. You can get coaching or assistance, but if you don't want to make the change, if you don't make that decision, you will not get better.

Thank you for your contribution. This conversation really sums up what we need to work on to improve our lifestyles. That is where we will leave the conversation—we have to put in the work in order to improve anything in our lives.

Summary and Review of Key Points

To finish up this book, I want to provide some key summaries and bullet points. Let's dive right in. Journaling is probably the most important component to understanding habits and what needs to be done to change those habits. Don't just start setting goals. Observe where you are now, then start making goals.

Journaling and Nutrition

Make sure to count everything while journaling what you eat. Work on initially understanding the number of calories you consume from processed sugar and carbohydrates. Reduce the number of calories that you intake by half and work to reduce meal portions. Next, work in an elimination/substitution diet. For example, exchange different types of high-calorie food sources to see how your body reacts, i.e. eliminate processed bread products and eat oats instead. This is where the N-of-1 Challenge is important. It will not be easy, it is a challenge! Next, sit down and plan two weeks of changes in your diet to start. It does not need to be perfect with the first try but you will eventually find your own optimized diet based on your needs. The elimination and substitution diet can be a fun experience as you learn how your body reacts to different types of foods.

Journaling and Core-Strength

Add a 15- to 20 -minute stretching regimen to your day. Work to perform some sort of activity for at least 45 minutes per day as well. Cardio and strength workouts do not need to be long to obtain the needed results. Mix different exercises to balance muscle groups. Make sure to journal your activities so that you can track data and plan goals. Plan time to sit down and review your data and plan. Besides the number of workouts per week, a valuable piece of data can be your heart rate while performing these workouts. Simply recording the number of steps you take in a day is a start, but not going to get you back to a healthy state.

Journaling and Mind-space

Your time is valuable, and you should work to eliminate negative influences. If you are overextended, take an inventory to determine what is important, otherwise classic burnout may be on the horizon. Sit down and journal different aspects of your life to determine your positive and negative influences. On a second form, also journal your positive and negative habits. This is where nutrition, core-strength, and mind-space meet. To be healthy, we need to manage all three aspects through being mindful of the positive and negative influences in all aspects of our lives.

Full Schedule and Personal Time

In this section, you will find a chart with days and times. Simply fill out your weekly schedule. The goal is to set aside time for yourself so that you can achieve new goals. Start by adding your everyday life items, then find times when workouts can be added. You may need to alter some of your everyday life items to make room for a workout. For me, if I put something on a schedule, I usually work hard to achieve it. If you are in a "re-start" phase, work to reclaim two hours of your week so that you can work towards a healthy lifestyle.

Coaches and Specialists

There is a coach or specialist for each of these important parts of our lives and they can be accessed individually as needed. The number of specialists and coaches that care about helping people is enormous. First, see your primary doctor — I prefer holistic-minded doctors. Ask questions about different types of specialists that you may be referred to so that you can have help forming a new habit. If you need a fitness coach, get a fitness coach. If you suffer from some sort of chronic pain that is not due to an acute injury, perhaps you need a mobility expert. Do you need a support group to help get through the difficult start-up time? There are groups and coaches for all types of people for all aspects of life. Your own N-of-1 Challenge will define where you need coaches and specialists.

Questions from Stories from Chapter 3

Below you will find the questions that we saw in Chapter 3 at the start of the book. What is your current story? This is another exercise to help you get started, or if you want to evaluate where you are now. Start putting your own N-of-1 Challenge goals down on paper. You can answer these questions to the best of your ability — there are no wrong answers. If there is a goal that you would like to reach under the heading, write it down. It does not need to be perfect the first time. What you write down now might change as you find your own N-of-1 Challenge.

Chart	Sunday	Monday	Tuesday	Wednesday	Thursday	Friday	Saturday
5:00 AM							
6:00 AM							
7:00 AM							
8:00 AM							
9:00 AM							
10:00 AM							
11:00 AM							
1:00 PM							
2:00 PM							
3:00 PM							
4:00 PM							
5:00 PM							
5:00 PM							
6:00 PM							
7:00 PM							
8:00 PM							
9:00 PM							

What is Your Personal N-of-1? The Reader.

1) While growing up, what sort of diet did you have, and what sorts of athletic activities did you participate in (high school through college)? Can you describe your diet from that time?

2) What were the factors (or reasons) that contributed to your loss in overall health?

3) What motivated you to become healthy again? Did you "wake up," or were you awake but did not act on what you knew you needed to do?

4) Are there specific fad diets/workouts that you tried that didn't work? Did you give up and restart several times, only to go back to being unhealthy?

5) Did you adopt any new meditative practices, power naps, or prayer schedules that helped "fill your cup" or "ease your mind"?

6) What is your final N-of-1 regimen for nutrition and physical activity, and how do you maintain the balance (mind-space) you have found? What does your diet now consist of? Do you have a system? (For example, 50% vegetables, 25% meat, 25% carbohydrates, etc.) What are your typical workouts or physical activities for the week? Do you have certain goals that you try to hit during the week?

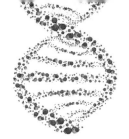

ABOUT
THE AUTHOR

Jeremiah Tipton grew up in the Tampa Bay area before moving to Melbourne, Florida for college at the Florida Institute of Technology. After receiving his Bachelor of Science in Research Chemistry, Jeremiah attended the University of Florida, Gainesville where he earned his Doctor of Philosophy in Bio-Analytical Chemistry. Following the completion of his degree, he has worked on numerous research projects

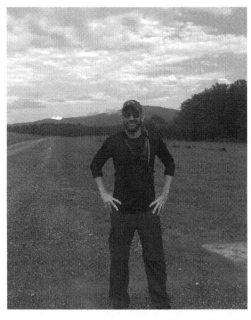

related to new drug discovery for different diseases and helped develop tests to define these diseases. Over the years, Jeremiah has become an expert in the field largely described as 'OMICS' - or understanding the systems, components, and biochemistry of molecular processes that work together to create life. Dr. Tipton has now developed a holistic, homeostatic view of the world with regards to health care and personal maintenance.

Currently, Jeremiah owns a consulting company working in the fields of OMICS Technology, Bio-Analytical Testing, and Next Generation Medical Tests. The next phase of Jeremiah's ambitions includes growing and sharing his story on how to look at nutrition, core-strength, and overall health. One of Dr. Tipton's passions is to have discussions on what types of diseases are avoidable. Our genetics is a great starting point for assessing a predisposition to a disease; but what about environmental and nutritional factors? What about factors that are within our control? Along with working in the field of Clinical Research, in the end, Jeremiah looks to make a difference in human health through basic education on nutrition, core-strength, and habit-forming behaviors.

APPENDICES

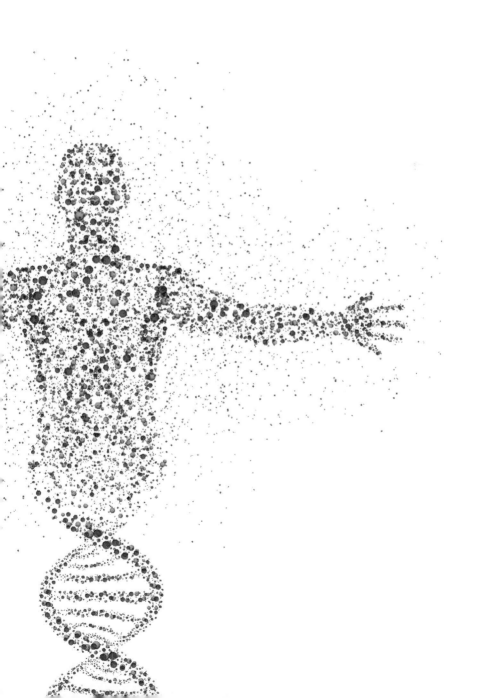

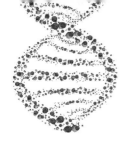

BIOGRAPHIES FOR THE SUBJECT MATTER EXPERTS

Dr. Alyssa Stewart

Alyssa is an owner, manager, and therapist at Empower PT. After graduating from the University of Florida with a degree in Exercise Physiology, she obtained a Doctorate in Physical Therapy from the University of Miami in 2009. Alyssa began working in both the outpatient and inpatient settings at St. Catherine's Rehabilitation Hospital, and quickly worked her way to Senior Physical Therapist. She then moved to South Tampa in 2011 where she served as a staff physical therapist for five years at St. Joseph's Hospital, working in both outpatient and inpatient rehab before deciding to open her own practice. Alyssa is committed to ongoing professional growth and frequently attends workshops and courses to improve her skills as a therapist. She is certified in Polestar Pilates for Rehabilitation, Selective Functional Movement Assessment (SFMA), Functional Movement Screen (FMS), Functional Range Conditioning (FRC), Titleist Performance Institute (TPI), full body Active Release Technique (ART), LSVT BIG for Parkinson's Disease, and is an APTA Clinical Educator for DPT students.

Dr. Dex Alvarez

Dr. Dex Alvarez is a third-generation Tampa native. Dr. Alvarez graduated from Jesuit High School in Tampa and earned his degree in Biological Science from Florida State University.

Soon after earning his bachelor's degree, Dr. Alvarez was accepted as one of only twelve students to be a part of the inaugural class of National University of Health Sciences Florida campus. Upon graduating with his Doctor of Chiropractic, Dr. Alvarez was also awarded the Joseph Janse Outstanding Graduate Award.

Dr. Alvarez is part of a larger group of chiropractors nationwide known as Maximized Living, whose purpose is to change and transform the way people view and manage their health care from the inside out. At their south Tampa location, the entire patient is given care. Dr. Alvarez not only provides spinal corrective care to his patients but also educates them on how to deal with everyday stresses by relaxing the mind, having proper nutrition, detoxifying the body, correcting spinal issues to allow proper nervous system function, and how to properly exercise to encourage optimum oxygenation to lean muscles.

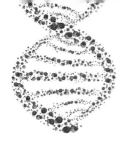

APPENDIX 2

SOME EXAMPLES OF STRETCHING AND FOAM ROLLING EXERCISES

Please note that this section provides some examples of stretches and exercises that you can perform . There are more stretches and exercises needed for a full regimen. Sources can be found on the internet as well as the www.nof1challenge.com website.

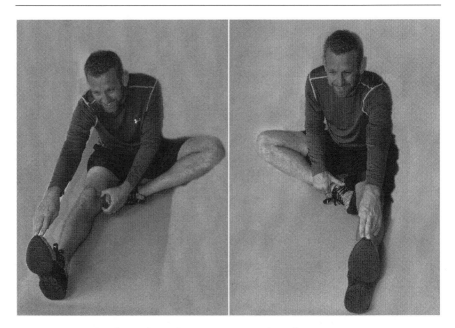

Figure 9 Example of Stretches - Sitting Hamstring Stretch

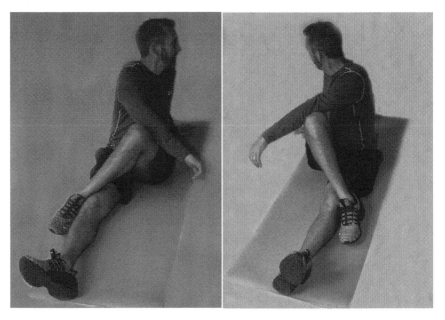

Figure 10 Example of Stretches - Back Stretch

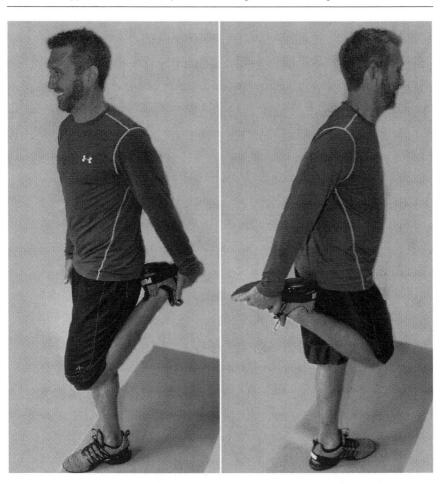

Figure 11 Example of Stretches - Standing Quad Stretch

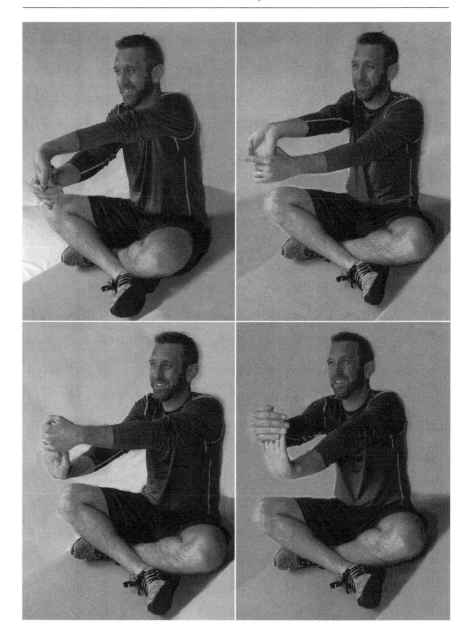

Figure 12 Example of Stretches - Simple Sitting Arm Stretch

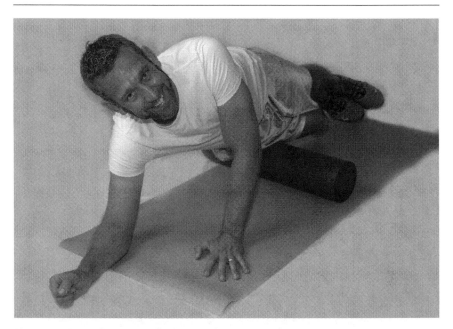

Figure 13 Example Foam Roller - IT Band

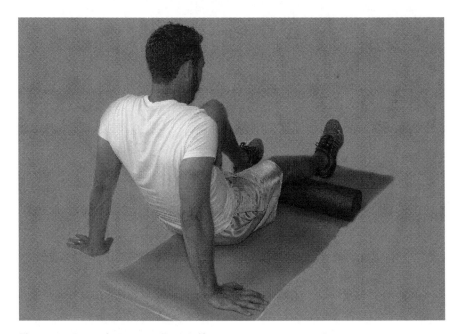

Figure 14 Example Foam Roller - Calf

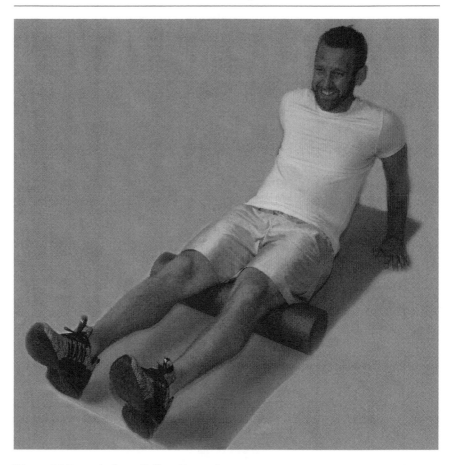

Figure 15 Example Foam Roller - Hamstring

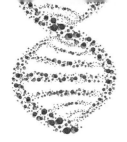

APPENDIX 3

SOME EXAMPLE EXERCISE TO PERFORM FOR CORE STRENGTH EXERCISES

Please note that this section provides some examples of exercises that you can perform without the need for expensive equipment or a gym membership. However, it is recommended that you join a gym or get a coach so that you can practice correct form. Also, there are more exercise needed for a full work out, including some of the base shown in this appendix.

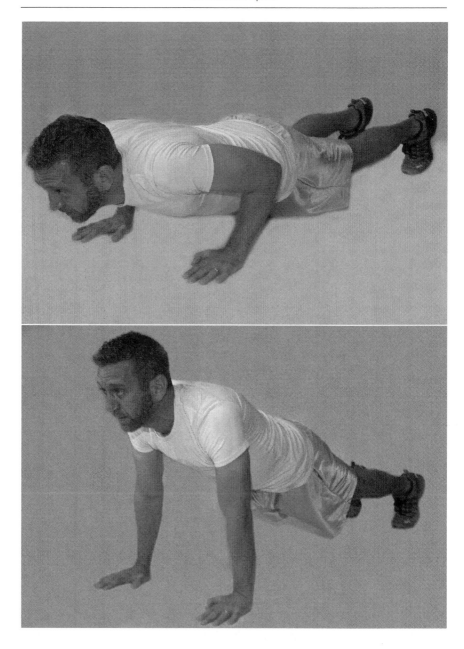

Figure 16 - Examples of Body Weight Workout Exercise - Common Push-Ups - Can add variety to this basic exercise.

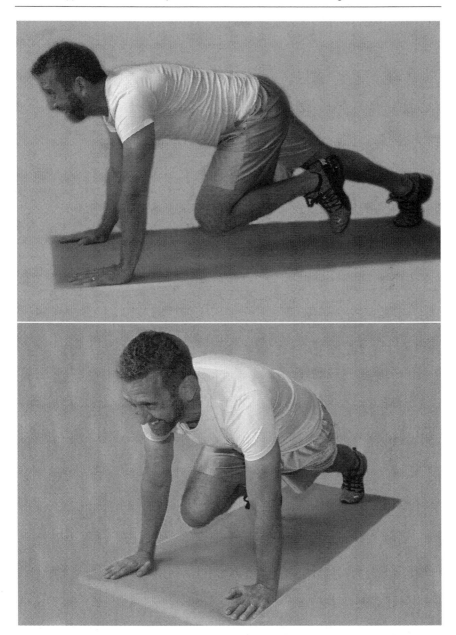

Figure 17 - Examples of Body Weight Workout Exercise - Mountain Climbers from Push-up Position - Can add variety to this basic exercise.

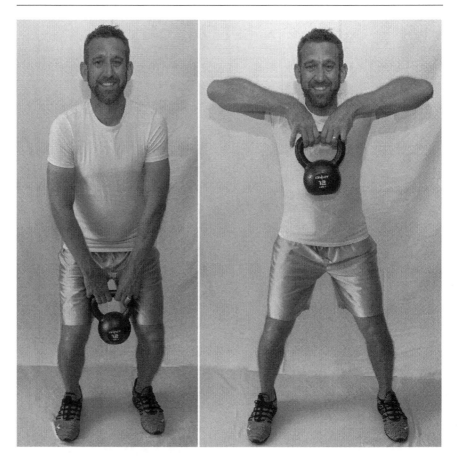

Figure 18 - Examples of Kettlebell Workout Exercise - Upright Row

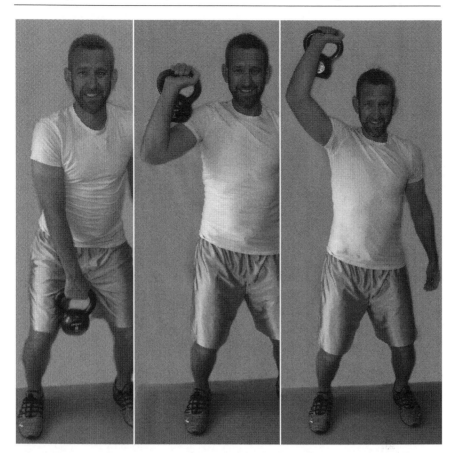

Figure 19 - Examples of Kettlebell Workout Exercise - Clean and Press Set for Right Side (Repeat for Left side as well)

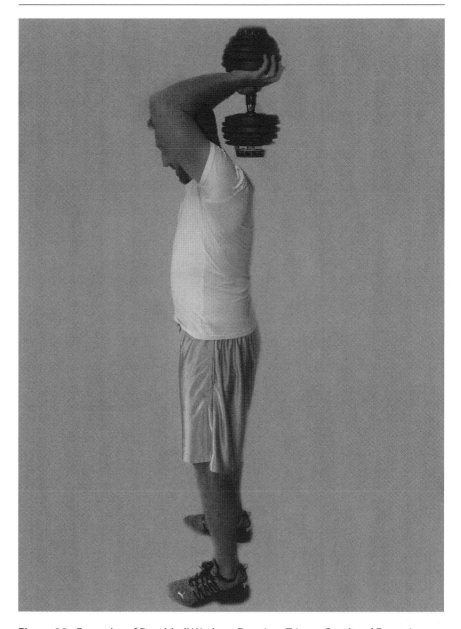

Figure 20 - Examples of Dumbbell Workout Exercise - Triceps Overhead Extension

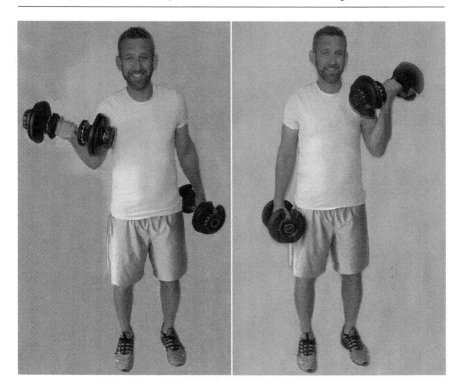

Figure 21 - Examples of Dumbbell Workout Exercise - Simple Bicep Curls

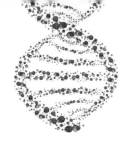

APPENDIX 4

REFERENCE LIST

REF 1 – The Power of Now: A Guide to Spiritual Enlightenment by Eckhart Tolle

REF 2 – The Power of Habit: Why We Do What We Do in Life and Business by Charles Duhigg

REF 3 – Mini Habits: Smaller Habits, Bigger Results by Stephen Guise

REF 4 - Nature ISSN 0028-0836 EISSN 1476-4687 Personalized medicine: Time for one-person trials. Nicholas J. Schork 29 April 2015 "Precision medicine requires a different type of clinical trial that focuses on individual, not average, responses to therapy, says Nicholas J. Schork."

REF 5 - [A]National Institute of Health: National Institute of Diabetes and Kidney Disease Diabetes Diet, Eating, & Physical Activity https://www.niddk.nih.gov/health-information/diabetes/overview/diet-eating-physical-activity

[B] American Diabetes Association. Foundations of care and comprehensive medical evaluation. Diabetes Care. 2016; 39 (suppl 1): S26 (Table 3.3).

[C] U.S. Department of Health and Human Services, Office of Disease Prevention and Health Promotion. 2008 Physical Activity Guidelines for Americans summary. https://health.gov/paguidelines/guidelines/summary.aspx. Updated June 21, 2016. Accessed June 21, 2016.

[E] Center for Disease Control and Prevention **REF 6** - Rethink Your Drink from the Centers for Disease Control and Prevention (CDC) https://www.cdc.gov/healthyweight/healthy_eating/drinks.html

REF 7 – The Food Addiction Paul J. Kenny Scientific American 309, 44 - 49 (2013) Published online: 20 August 2013doi:10.1038/scientificamerican0913-44 https://www.nature.com/scientificamerican/journal/v309/n3/box/scientificamerican0913-44_BX1.html

REF 8 –Is Food Addiction Making Us Fat? Paul J. Kenny Scientific America June 2015 Volume 24, Issue 2s https://www.scientificamerican.com/article/is-food-addiction-making-us-fat/

REF 9 - UCSF - the Sugar Science group How Much Is Too Much? The growing concern over too much added sugar in our diets. http://sugarscience.ucsf.edu/the-growing-concern-of-overconsumption.html#.XAlGgHRKg2w

REF 10 - Harvard Medical School (HMS) glycemic index for over 60+ foods https://www.health.harvard.edu/diseases-and-conditions/glycemic-index-and-glycemic-load-for-100-foods

REF 11 - Harvard T.H. Chan School of Public Health – The Nutrition Source https://www.hsph.harvard.edu/nutritionsource/carbohydrates/carbohydrates-and-blood-sugar/

REF 12 - "International tables of glycemic index and glycemic load values: 2008" by Fiona S. Atkinson, Kaye Foster-Powell, and Jennie C. Brand-Miller in the December 2008 issue of Diabetes Care, Vol. 31, number 12, pages 2281-2283.

REF 13 - U.S. Department of Health & Human Services; National Heart, Lung, and Blood Institute. Healthy Weight Tools. https://www.nhlbi.nih.gov/health/educational/lose_wt/BMI/index.htm https://www.nhlbi.nih.gov/health/educational/lose_wt/risk.htm

REF 14 - Center for Disease Control and Prevention. About Adult BMI https://www.cdc.gov/healthyweight/assessing/bmi/adult_bmi/index.html

REF 15 - National Institute of Diabetes and Digestive and Kidney Diseases Health Information Center. Risk Factors for Type 2 Diabetes. https://www.niddk.nih.gov/health-information/diabetes/overview/risk-factors-type-2-diabetes

REF 16 - United States Department of Agriculture, Center for Nutrition Policy and Promotion. https://www.cnpp.usda.gov/ Estimated Calorie Needs per Day by Age, Gender, and Physical Activity Level https://www.cnpp.usda.gov/sites/default/files/usda_food_patterns/ EstimatedCalorieNeedsPerDayTable.pdf

REF 17 - American Heart Association - Added Sugars http://www. heart.org/en/healthy-living/healthy-eating/eat-smart/sugar/ added-sugars.

REF 18 - [A] The University of San Francisco Sugar Science, The Un Sweet tooth. http://sugarscience.ucsf.edu/the-growing-concern-of-over-consumption.html#.XC-vElxKg2x

[B] - American Heart Association – Information on Sugar http://www. heart.org/en/healthy-living/healthy-eating/eat-smart/sugar/ added-sugars

REF 19 - The Conversation, A history of sugar – the food nobody needs, but everyone craves Mark Horton Professor in Archaeology, UnI of Bristol; Alexander BentIessor and Chair of Comparative Cultural Studies, University of Houston; Philip LangtonSenior Teaching Fellow in Physiology, University of Bristol October 30, 2015 https://theconversation.com/a-history-of-sugar-the-food-nobody-needs-but-everyone-craves-49823

REF 20 - Average Person Consumes 300% more Sugar Daily than 'Recommended'. Natural Society, Transforming your health naturally BY ELIZABETH RENTER. JANUARY 16, 2013. http://naturalsociety.com/ sugar-the-toxicity-question-and-what-to-do-about-it/

REF 21 - AHA Scientific Statement. Dietary Sugars Intake and Cardiovascular Health. A Scientific Statement from the American Heart Association. Circulation. 2009;120:1011-1020

REF 22 - Online Statistics Education: An Interactive Multimedia Course of Study Created by Rice University (Lead Ir), University of Houston Clear Lake, and Tufts University Chapter 20: Case Studies, Sugar Consumption in us Diets.

REF 23 - By 2606, the US Diet will be 100 Percent Sugar by Stephen Guyenet and Jeremy Laden data. February 18, 2012 Whole Health Source

- Nutrition and Health Science http://wholehealthsource.blogspot.com/2012/02/by-2606-us-diet-will-be-100-percent.html

REF 24 - "Sugar Rush! How Sugar Consumption is Changing America" An Accel Research Site https://www.avail-clinical.com/news/sugar-rush-how-sugar-consumption-is-changing-america-infographic/

REF 25 - Statistics About Diabetes. American Diabetes Association. Overall Numbers, Diabetes and Prediabetes. http://www.diabetes.org/diabetes-basics/statistics/

REF 26 - From the National Institute of Diabetes and Digestive and Kidney Disease https://www.niddk.nih.gov/health-information/health-statistics/overweight-obesity

REF 27 - US Department of Health and Human Services – National Institute of Health Eunice Kennedy Shriver National Institute of Child Health and Human Development Health Research throughout the lifespan - What causes diabetes? https://www.nichd.nih.gov/health/topics/diabetes/conditioninfo/causes#f3

REF 28 - The Mayo Clinic - Patient Car & Health Information - Diseases & Conditions - Diabetes https://www.mayoclinic.org/diseases-conditions/diabetes/symptoms-causes/syc-20371444

REF 29 - Arch Pharm Res. 2013 Feb;36(2):201-7. doi: 10.1007/s12272-013-0020-y. Epub 2013 Jan 29. Molecular mechanisms of central leptin resistance in obesity. Jung CH1, Kim MS

REF 30 - National Institute of Diabetes and Digestive and Kidney Disease. Diabetes Overview - Risk Factors for Type 2 Diabetes https://www.niddk.nih.gov/health-information/diabetes/overview/risk-factors-type-2-diabetes

REF 31 - American Diabetes Association. What We Recommend http://www.diabetes.org/food-and-fitness/fitness/types-of-activity/what-we-recommend.html

REF 32 - [A] National Institute of Health: National Institute of Diabetes and Kidney Disease Diabetes Diet, Eating, & Physical Activity https://www.niddk.nih.gov/health-information/diabetes/overview/diet-eating-physical-activity

[B] American Diabetes Association. Foundations of care and comprehensive medical evaluation. Diabetes Care. 2016;39(suppl 1): S26 (Table 3.3).

[C] U.S. Department of Health and Human Services, Office of Disease Prevention and Health Promotion. 2008 Physical Activity Guidelines for Americans summary. https://health.gov/paguidelines/guidelines/summary.aspx Updated June 21, 2016. Accessed June 21, 2016.

REF 33 - U.S. Department of Health & Human Services. National Institutes of Health. Human Microbiome Project, https://commonfund.nih.gov/hmp

REF 34 – [A] Strains, functions and dynamics in the expanded Human Microbiome Project. Lloyd-Price, J.; Mahurkar, A.; Rahnavard, G.; Crabtree, J.;Orvis, J.; Hall, A.B.; Brady, A.; Creasy, H.H.; McCracken C.; Giglio, M.G.; McDonald, D.; Franzosa, EA; Knight, R,; White, O. Huttenhower. Nature. 2017 Oct 5;550(7674):61-66. doi: 10.1038/nature23889. Epub 2017 Sep 20.

[B] Structure, function and diversity of the healthy human microbiome. Human Microbiome Project Consortium. Numerous Authors Nature. 2012 Jun 13;486(7402):207-14. doi: 10.1038/nature11234.

[C] The Integrative Human Microbiome Project: dynamic analysis of microbiome-host omics profiles during periods of human health and disease. Integrative HMP (iHMP) Research Network Consortium. Cell Host Microbe. 2014 Sep 10;16(3):276-89. doi: 10.1016/j.chom.2014.08.014.

[D] The gut mycobiome of the Human Microbiome Project healthy cohort. Nash, A.K.; Auchtung, T.A.; Wong M.C.; Smith D.P.; Gesell, J.R.; Ross, M.C.; Stewart, C.J.; Metcalf, G.A.; Muzny, D.M.; Gibbs, R.A.; Ajami, N.J.; Petrosino, J.F. Microbiome. 2017 Nov 25;5(1):153. doi: 10.1186/s40168-017-0373-4.

REF 35 - Mind-Body Connection Therapies by Merrily A. Kuhn, RN, Ph.D.

Made in the USA
Columbia, SC
06 July 2019